The Père Marquette
Lecture in Theology
2004

Bioethics and
the Common Good

Lisa Sowle Cahill

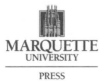

MARQUETTE
UNIVERSITY
PRESS

Library of Congress Cataloging-in-Publication Data
Cahill, Lisa Sowle.
Bioethics and the common good / Lisa Sowle Cahill.
    p. cm. — (The Père Marquette lecture in theology ;
2004)
    ISBN 0-87462-584-X (cloth bound : alk. paper)
    1. Bioethics—Religious aspects—Catholic Church.
I. Title. II. Series.
    QH332.C344 2004
    241'.64957—dc22

                                        2004001874

© 2004
Marquette University Press
Milwaukee WI 53201-3141
All rights reserved.

Manufactured in the United States of America
Member, Association of American University Presses

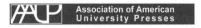

MARQUETTE UNIVERSITY PRESS
MILWAUKEE

The Association of Jesuit University Presses

Foreword

This year's Père Marquette Lecture in Theology marks the thirtieth-fourth lecture in the series, inaugurated in 1969 to commemorate the missions and explorations of Père Jacques Marquette, S.J. (1637-75). Held annually under the auspices of Marquette University's Department of Theology, it continues to be funded generously by the Joseph A. Auchter Family Endowment Fund, named after Milwaukee-native Joseph A. Auchter (1894-1986), a banker, paper-industry executive, and long-time supporter of education. The fund was established by his children as a memorial to their father.

Lisa Sowle Cahill

This year's lecturer is Lisa Sowle Cahill, a central figure in contemporary Roman Catholic moral theology, and indeed a central figure in the broader field of Christian Ethics. Dr. Cahill received her B.A. in Theology from Santa Clara University in 1970, followed by M.A. and Ph.D. degrees from the University of Chicago Divinity School, where she wrote her dissertation under the supervision of James Gustafson (1976). She is J. Donald Monan, S.J., Professor in the Department of Theology at Boston College, where she has taught since 1976, and has been a Visiting Scholar at the Kennedy Institute of Ethics, Georgetown University (1986) and Visiting Professor of Catholic Theology at Yale University (1997).

Dr. Cahill is a fellow of the American Academy of Arts and Sciences, and has held office in the American Academy of Religion. She has served as an editor, or on the editorial boards, of *Concilium*, *Journal of Religious Ethics*, *Interpretation: A Journal of Bible and Theology*, *Religious Studies Review*, *Journal of Medicine and Philosophy*, *Horizons*, *Journal of Law and Religion*, *Second Opinion*, and the *Kennedy Institute of Ethics Journal*. In addition, she has been a member of the Catholic Health Association Theology and Ethics Advisory Committee, the National Advisory Board for Ethics in Reproduction, and serves on the March of Dimes National Bioethics Committee. She has given testimony to the National Bioethics Advisory Commission on fetal tissue research and on cloning. For five years she convened a small international study group on genetics, theology, and social ethics.

Special areas of interest from among her many areas of expertise areas are fundamental theological ethics, the use of Scripture in ethics, the ethics of sex and gender, bioethics, just war theory and pacifism, and history of Christian ethics. A current research focus is genetics and social ethics, including cloning, stem cell research, and the international development and marketing of genomics-based tests and therapies. Another interest is challenges to, applications of, and alternatives to, Christian just war theory today.

These areas of specialization are represented in her many publications. She has written or edited eight books, with a ninth in progress: *Family: A Christian Social Perspective* (Fortress, 2000); *Sex, Gender, and Christian Ethics* (Cambridge University Press, 1996); *"Love Your Enemies": Discipleship, Pacifism, and Just War Theory* (Fortress, 1994); *Between the Sexes: Toward a Christian Ethics of Sexuality* (Fortress and Paulist Presses, 1985); *Women and Sexuality* (Paulist, 1992); and, with Thomas A. Shannon, *Religion and Artificial Reproduction: An Inquiry into the Vatican Instruction on Human Life* (Crossroad Press, 1988); *Embodiment, Morality and Medicine* with Margaret A. Farley (Kluwer Publishers, 1995), and, with James Childress, *Christian Ethics: Problems and Prospects*, a collection in honor of James M. Gustafson (Pilgrim Press, 1996). Currently she is preparing for publication an edited volume called *Genetics, Theology, Ethics: An Interdisciplinary Conversation* (Crossroad). She is the author of approximately 150 essays that have appeared in books or in journals such as *Theological Studies, Journal of Religion, Journal of Religious Ethics, Hastings Center Report, Journal of Medicine and Philosophy, Kennedy Institute of Ethics Journal, Journal of Law and Religion, Law, Medicine, and Health Care, Hofstra Law Review, Loyola Law Review, Horizons, Interpretation, Thought*, and *Concilium*.

On its own it is a great honor for Marquette's Department of Theology to have a lecturer of the accomplishment and esteem of Lisa Sowle Cahill.

But her lecturing in our series has a fittingness that goes beyond the appropriateness of having so central an individual in contemporary Catholic moral theology address us on a topic of great importance; for, as it happens, in giving the Père Marquette Lecture this year Dr. Cahill will be following in the footsteps of two previous lecturers in this series, from whom she is an intellectual descendent: James M. Gustafson (1975), who directed her dissertation, and Richard A. McCormick, S.J., (1973), who figured prominently in her dissertation, and in her work thereafter. We thank her for addressing us on "Bioethics and the Common Good," and contributing this volume to posterity in our midst, fully expecting that it will be found on the bookshelf of some future Père Marquette Lecturer.

Mark F. Johnson
March 21, 2004

Bioethics and the Common Good

Lisa Sowle Cahill

In 1973 and 1975, Marquette Theology Lectures with subject matter similar to mine were delivered by my two most important theological mentors: the Protestant theologian James M. Gustafson (1975), who was then my dissertation director at the University of Chicago; and Richard A. McCormick, S.J. (1973), to whom Gustafson introduced me, and whose work became a central part of my dissertation. The little blue volumes bearing the names of these theological "greats" have been treasured items on my library shelf for many years. Imagine my delight and trepidation at being invited to make a contribution to the same series three decades later. Though neither as original in content nor as forceful in style as the lectures of my teachers, my own bears testimony to their influence and to the importance of ecumenical conversation in the development of Catholic tradition.[1] The Marquette Theology Lectures have for decades been a sponsor of thoughtful, creative dialogue among Catholics and between Catholics and Protestants.

One goal of my lecture will be to show how Catholic moral theology, especially as focused on decisions about preserving life and enhancing health, is changing in its perspectives, methods, and characteristic emphases, in response to the challenges and opportunities of what we now call "globalization." Globalization is bringing Catholic bioethics ever more firmly under the aegis of Catholic social teaching and the common good, without, however, losing its characteristic emphasis on the dignity and inviolability of the individual person.

The common good defines a solidaristic association of persons that is more than the good of individuals in the aggregate. "Common good" says something about social communication and cooperation as essential to the fulfillment of our very personhood. The notion of common good is central to the Catholic social tradition, but it did not really begin its migration to Catholic medical ethics until well after the middle of the twentieth century. As we open the twenty-first century, the orientation of Catholic bioethics is different than it was for the greater part of the twentieth. The very term "*bio*ethics" expands our vision to life and health outside the delimited context of healthcare facilities and "medical" interventions. It even suggests that human life is and should be integrated with all life and the entire natural environment. Individual life and health now must be seen in the perspective of the common good—not just of the family, local community, province, nation, region, or continent, but of all human societies and of life on the planet.

The Catholic concept of the common good has always tied person and society together by insisting that the intrinsic sociality of persons demands their interdependence, communication, solidarity, and co-responsibility.[2] Especially since the pontificate of John XXIII, the common good has been construed as globally comprehensive. Moreover, the participation of all persons and groups in institutions of decision-making has been affirmed, and the "preferential option for the poor" has been proclaimed as a Christian and social duty. This perspective of modern Catholic social teaching is transforming what used to be called "medical ethics." Bioethics is now appreciated to be a variety of social ethics, in which an ever greater concern is patterns of access to health care. Not only do many in our own country lack health insurance, but millions around the world lack the ability to meet basic needs, and suffer from devastating illnesses like tuberculosis, malaria, and AIDS.

After having traced the development of social bioethics over the last three decades, beginning with the Marquette lectures of McCormick and Gustafson, I will turn my attention to a current and quite significant problem for Catholic bioethics as an ethics of the common good: practicability. It will come as news to few of my hearers or readers that Catholic bioethics has the newly energized social focus I have described, or that religious leaders and theologians are looking beyond national health care reform to urge responsibility for global health inequities. Now we need to "problematize" the bioethics of the common good as a practical agenda. Can a "bioethics of the common good" make any difference in the real world? I believe it can. I will use the AIDS crisis to show that a bioethics of the common good is already being put into practice. An impressive variety of local and mid-level, as well as national and transnational, institutions, many operating under Catholic auspices, are mobilizing to fight AIDS.

McCormick and Gustafson

The question of a social bioethics is clearly present in James Gustafson's Marquette Lecture. Here he was ahead of Catholic thinkers of the same era. Yet for McCormick as well, the social dimensions of bioethics are implicit, even though the starting point of his 1973 Marquette Lecture was norms for individual decision-making. A contrast with Gustafson will help to highlight some distinctively "Catholic" aspects of McCormick's thought, both in regard to what he values and in regard to what he omits.

Unlike theological authors prior to the 1960's, who might have tended to present their views as timelessly objective and standpoint-free pronouncements about God and "man," both McCormick and

Gustafson are careful to allude to their locations within particular theological traditions, and to note the historical development of same. For Gustafson, the Christian tradition provides a "theological moral point of view" in which all human endeavors must be placed under the sovereignty of God, the ultimate power. Gustafson emphasizes that the purposes of God include the well-being of the entire creation, not of humanity alone.[3] He proposes that the concept of the "common good" be extended beyond the good of particular human communities such as families or nations, and even beyond the human race as such. "It becomes necessary to think of the good of plants and water, air and minerals, as well as the good of human communities."[4] Gustafson then raises the possibility that moral judgments will be necessary that "override certain human claims for individual rights and values for the sake of the more inclusive well-being of a wider circle of life." Human beings may be distinctive, but they are not the pinnacle of creation; the needs and interests of the species, as is even more true of individuals, should not be absolutized over the well-being of the creation "of which the human is but a part."[5]

Gustafson never tries to set up a clear hierarchy of the value of beings, or establish ordering principles to determine how to resolve conflicts among values. Instead, he sees the contributions of theology to a moral point of view to consist primarily in theology's affirmation of the reality of God. Secondarily, the-

ology establishes certain attitudes or dispositions
to guide moral discernment, such as responsibility,
openness to change, and self-criticism deriving from
acknowledgment of fallibility and sin. Values are
plural and they may conflict, as happens frequently in
medical research and care.[6] Hence decisions must be
made in light of relationships involved in a particular
case; risk is almost always part of the picture; and
"absolute moral certitude is impossible."[7] It seems
that for Gustafson, one of the main "contributions
of theology to medial ethics" is to remind decision-
makers of the inescapable fact of "ambiguity in
moral choice."

Though this was actually Richard McCormick's
title,[8] ambiguity was a subject he approached much
more tentatively than Gustafson, and within a
much narrower range. McCormick's lecture was not
directly on medical ethics, but it engaged a principle
key to Catholic thought in this area, the principle
of double effect.[9] The idea behind this principle is
that people can find themselves in moral situations in
which a compelling good can be achieved only at the
price of causing some evil (the "double" effect). The
principle provides that the evil effect can be tolerated
as long as the act in question is not already "intrinsically evil in itself," the good is greater, the evil is not
directly "intended" or wanted for its own sake, the
evil effect is not directly caused by the action in a
physical sense, and the evil effect is not the means
to the good one.[10] Long a staple of Catholic moral

theology, this principle had been used (and still is) to try to eliminate virtually all ambiguity from choices in some of the most difficult areas of human life and death, including just war, abortion, and ending life-prolonging medical treatment.

Though raising questions about the certitude this principle was thought to guarantee, McCormick certainly still shared with traditional moral theology the ideas that there is an objective morality based on an objective order of values that is not inherently conflictual. McCormick also agreed with Catholic tradition that some actions are intrinsically wrong, and that any ambiguity attending choice is more a matter of human epistemological limits than of glitches and gaps in the "real" moral universe. From this perspective, conflict is due to sin, not God's ordering of things. But McCormick did not believe that God allows sin to create ultimate conflicts among the most important values, moral values (states of character and of intersubjective relationship, such as truthfulness, fidelity and love).[11]

Nevertheless, McCormick's title calls attention to the "ambiguity" that so often attends the application of traditional moral principles and rules to concrete situations and choices. In his introductory remarks, McCormick grants that "the rule of double effect has had an honored and very important place in the formulation of Catholic moral theology and teaching." Nevertheless, he continues, there have recently been "rumblings of dissatisfaction, uncertainty, disagreement—or all three." Some critics had tried "to test its traditional understanding, to challenge its decisiveness, or even to deny its moral relevance."[12]

Without a doubt, the explorations McCormick engaged at Marquette arose from controversies over the morality of individual actions in two key areas, sexual behavior and medical decisions, areas which often overlapped. Contraception, abortion, and the new reproductive technologies are illustrative. McCormick delivered his lecture in the year of the *Roe v. Wade* abortion decision, five years after the publication of *Humanae vitae*, and five years prior to the birth of the first "test-tube baby," Louise Brown. McCormick also wrote at a time of great controversy over the use of medical technologies in end-of-life care. In the United States, an active pro-euthanasia movement found a vocal spokesperson in Derek Humphry, head of the Hemlock Society, who advocated mercy-killing as a necessary way to protect "death with dignity" and to avoid the prolonged captivity of terminal patients in high-tech intensive care units.[13] Only a few years before McCormick's lecture, the Second Vatican Council had acclaimed openness to the modern world, called upon the expertise of lay people, and urged the renewal of moral theology. Clearly, McCormick was prompted by contemporary moral quandaries and by voices calling for change to probe the premises and principles of the moral theology in which he had been educated.

McCormick arrived at the conclusion, shared by other moralists of the time (such as Josef Fuchs, Bruno Schüller, and Peter Knauer) that objective moral knowledge can be best attained by taking carefully into consideration all the details of moral situations. It is not enough to apply abstract rules to "actions," the definitions of which are truncated through elimination of circumstances, and whose moral character has been prejudged. His corollary points were that the principle of double effect, as traditionally interpreted, does not furnish the certainty it promises as a guide to moral objectivity, and that, moreover, its conditions are internally incoherent. He claimed, for instance, that the key to the principle was the proportion of good over bad, and that the requirement that the evil effect not be the path to the good had no clear rationale. Moreover, if the good outweighs the bad, it can be fairly assumed that the intention is directed to the good as the goal of the action; so-called "indirectness" of action as well as of intention is not necessary to guarantee the agent's rectitude. Most controversially, McCormick and others argued that the category of "intrinsically evil acts," by which some actions were totally precluded from any possible justification, even by double effect, was incoherent. They contended that some actions (especially contraception) were placed in this category without full consideration of contingencies that could change the act's moral character.[14] With all these caveats, however, McCormick renounced neither the objectivity of moral values in general, nor the absolute moral value of the individual human being and his or her spiritual and moral character. Here he differed from, and was much less radical than, Gustafson, whose subsequent Marquette Lecture constitutes a reprimand of moral theology's self-assurance.

Of course, McCormick was still concerned to acknowledge and identify a space for ambiguity as endemic to practical moral reasoning. Where is that window of "ambiguity" for McCormick? And, in light of my larger project to connect bioethics to the common good, how does this window open onto morality's social context? For McCormick and other "proportionalists" the moral character of an act derives primarily and ultimately from the good intended by the agent: is the good intended and sought in fact the highest good at stake in the concrete circumstances of decision, as far as the agent can ascertain? Ambiguity occurs at two levels, at least. First, there can be ambiguity in the determination of *what is* the highest good in a conflict situation. Although given the objectivity of morals, it must be possible to compare and rank goods, human knowledge is limited, and the process of analysis tentative and imprecise. Thus determination of whether or not proportionate reason exists for an evil-producing action can be vexing and inconclusive.

Second, and related, McCormick is committed to affirm the equal value of every person, and the undeniable value of all persons, even in decisions where causing evil to some is tolerated as an outcome. Therefore another area of ambiguity concerns the possibly utilitarian or consequentialist implications of proportionate reason as the main provision of double effect. McCormick is not arguing that morality is defined simply as the "greatest good for the greatest number," maintaining like Gustafson that the needs and interests of some persons may have to be overridden in the process. McCormick is still part of the traditional universe of Catholic moral theology in which irresolvable conflicts of moral values are only apparent, not real. The distance of McCormick's position from Gustafson's is evident in his statement that, "I believe in a providential God in whose world the conflicts we experience do have a resolution."[15] No genuinely required moral choice could entail the violation of some individuals' genuine rights or dignity. So a second area of ambiguity, then, is the relation between proportionate reason, especially as concerning the "common good" of more than one person; and the value of *every* person to be affected by a decision, especially ones bearing the brunt of an evil effect. The problem is that it may seem difficult or impossible to further the common good of all, while giving every individual equal rights.

Proportionate Reason and Proportionalism

McCormick looks for ways to separate proportionalism from utilitarianism or consequentialism, though his efforts in this direction (and those of similar thinkers) have never been fully successful. In *Ambiguity in Moral Choice*, and later writings, McCormick keeps probing the notion of proportionate reason, trying to define it in such a way that it is consistent both with equal respect and with some absolute moral norms. In *Ambiguity in Moral Choice*, he denies that "proportionate reason is reducible to a simple utilitarian calculus." Trying to clarify this point, he says that "the notion of proportionate reason is analogous."[16] By saying that proportionate reason is analogous, McCormick means that the "good" toward which proportionate reasoning is directed may be understood in at least three different but similar ways. These are: the good of avoiding some greater evil; the good of justice as allowing self-preservation as the agent's priority; and gospel identity as prioritizing love and self-sacrifice for another, even at cost to the agent. All of these may be valid ways to resolve a moral problem. These three determinations of the "greater good" are forms of proportionate reason, but "the good" sought can validly be defined in three different ways, allowing for different acceptable outcomes. This proposal turns out to be very useful in understanding and applying the relevance of the notion of common good for bioethics in an era of globalization.

Essentially, the method of analogous reasoning from case to case is a way of introducing considerations of context and specificity into moral discernment, without giving up either the ideal of objective moral analysis or the acknowledgment that standpoints, perceptions, and needs are relative.[17] More importantly, it allows moral considerations that were originally applied in the contexts of single agents and their actions to be extended "analogously" to groups and institutions whose behavior occurs in larger patterns and networks that overlap, intersect, and extend over time. Globalization requires that we think of the good in different ways too. The "common good" globally requires at least three different approaches built on the ones McCormick has named. The global common good demands that "first world" nations avoid the greater evil of self-benefiting institutions that cause harm to others ("structural violence"), even if this means accepting the "lesser evil" of not maximizing their own opportunities for scientific and economic advancement. The global common good demands that we seek basic justice for all, but any nation or people is allowed to put its needs first, as long as it does not offend against the legitimate rights of others. The global common good also requires that we recognize the Christian vocation of self-sacrifice and preferential option for the poor as necessary for social transformation, going beyond rights and equality. These are different, complementary elements of global justice that may be appropriate in different contexts, and they are analogous to the ways individual decision-makers choose the lesser evil, have a right to self-preservation, and sometimes act altruistically to further the welfare of others.

In a recent article entitled, "Where have All the Proportionalists Gone?," Aline Kalbian argues that, though literature of the last decade has not continued to debate the merits of this so-called theory (which I believe is more a loose category of types of criticism than "a" constructive theory), McCormick at al. were neither defeated by counterarguments nor silenced by the *magisterium*. Rather, their concerns have transmuted into other sorts of literature, including revised natural law thinking, feminist thinking, and virtue theory. According to Kalbian, proportionalism "was motivated by concerns about seeing moral action in a more contextual way", a way "more attentive to particularity and moral agency."[18] Her thesis is "that proportionalism cleared out a conceptual space that has encouraged a hospitable atmosphere for these more particularistic approaches."[19]

While I believe Kalbian is right in this claim, I would push it a little further. If context and particularity are taken seriously, it quickly becomes evident that agents and their "virtues" are never isolated selves, nor are "acts" analyzable purely "in themselves," or even "in context," without reference to the discourses, varieties of social ethos, and institutions of practical and political life that shape the identities and opportunities of agents. The questions raised by proportionalism very rapidly open the door to the realization that all "personal" ethics, or ethics of agency, virtue and vice, are ineluctably also social ethics. Kalbian nearly says as much when she observes that proportionalism's teleological foundations and construction of moral agency share important elements with "the Thomistic ideal of the 'common good.'"[20]

One reason that the language and the original controversies of proportionalism have not continued to grip the interest of moral theologians with the same tenacity with which they controlled debates of thirty years ago is that the conceptual framework that generated the debate is not adequate to understand, much less to complete, the paradigm shifts proportionalism precipitated. The originating framework was double effect, a model primarily of individual decision-making about separate acts. One shift away from this moral worldview occurred when the proportionalists looked toward the agent more than the act. Still another occurred insofar as they worked with a much more contextual understanding of agency. A third shift came about when developers of the proportionalist critique, such as feminist and liberation theologians, realized that ethics of acts and agency must be integrated with political, institutional, and social ethics. The framework of "double effect," even in revised form, was unable to make this leap. Thus, since the 1980's, Catholic ethicists have turned increasingly to the resources of Thomistic ethics (premodern and community-focused) and of modern Catholic social teaching, even in taking up issues of sexual and medical ethics.

McCormick's discussion of proportionate reason shows at one and the same time the excitement and fertility of the new questions raised, and the limits of the manualist paradigm of an act-oriented moral theology. McCormick's critique never directly challenged this paradigm. The conditions of double effect still controlled the discussion of "proportionalism" for both its proponents and its opponents. Even while objecting to the category "intrinsically evil acts," McCormick sought ways to understand the morality of acts in an "intrinsic" way. Yet he peppered his discussion with examples (e.g., war and its social roots and effects) that clearly escaped the tools and focus "double effect" provided.

One reason for McCormick's abiding interest in defining morality in terms of characteristics intrinsic to certain specific types of action was that he could see as well as his critics that if the morality of individual decisions were too loosely tied to broad or long-range social considerations, the dangers of utilitarianism and fascism lurked not far away. And even at close range, too one-sidedly "contextual" an interpretation of moral responsibility would make it difficult to sustain at the practical level the commitment to "objective" morality that was espoused at the theoretical. Therefore, McCormick, of a mindset quite similar to his critics, never lost his desire to reconnect "contextuality"—quickly catapulting far beyond the horizon of the principle of double effect—to the interior, intrinsic, and clearly explicable character of individual acts. On another level, however, he realized that with "proportionate reason" he had sent up a trial balloon that would change the landscape of moral theology forever.

Further Consideration of Proportionate Reason, Moral Judgment, and Social Context

Briefly recapitulated, then, McCormick shows that proportionate reason can refer to at least three things: avoid the greater evil; perform a supererogatory altruistic act; or make the choice natural justice indicates, even if self-preservation will mean forfeiting the opportunity to save another. In other words, this criterion presents us with the prospect that the right and good act can be more than one of a number of things, even though there is an objective ranking of moral goods.[21] Proportionate reason is "analogous" and non-univocal in meaning. McCormick's explanation is good as far as it goes, but it also raises questions it does not resolve. It implicitly attributes conflicts individuals face at least in part to their social context, but does not sustain attention to this context when proposing resolutions. To be specific, the examples McCormick gives in *Ambiguity in Moral Choice* (e.g., saving a drowning swimmer and abortion) envision primarily one agent's choice in regard to another individual. Yet the entire discussion of these choices presupposes a

world of conflict, brokenness and sin that make such
choices necessary. After all, in an ideal world, one's
own life and welfare would not in any way conflict
with the needs of other persons. The broken social
conditions of choice are especially clear when we
consider all the factors that drive desperate women to
seek abortions. In a prelapsarian, undisrupted world,
there would be need neither for avoiding "greater
evils," nor for Christian exhortations to altruism,
since there would be neither conflicts nor any bias
of self-interest turning us away from the good of
others. Social relations and institutionalized patterns
of behavior would all coincide perfectly with the
well-being of every individual and of the common
good. The fundamental cause of the conflicts and
ambiguities faced by individual moral agents is the
disordered character of the world they live in and
the social practices in which we all participate. Yet
there is a gap between McCormick's presupposition
of social disorder as conditioning hard choices and
his focus (like traditional double effect) on individual
decision-making.

The missing element seems to me to be attention
to the way social structures mediate brokenness and
conflict. Distorted structures and social practices
can force even the virtuous agent to make choices
that reflect the brokenness of the choice's social
context. Worse, distorted structures create bias in
agents by reinforcing attitudes and priorities that
are then "rationalized" through misapplied moral

constructs. John T. Ford's brilliant article on the immorality of obliteration bombing in World War II grasped this point very clearly.[22] He charged moralists and politicians with misapplying double effect so that the deaths of civilians brought about by the bombing of whole cities could be termed "indirect" collateral damage. The policy of obliteration bombing was part of a whole moral-political ethos that absolutized the Allies' determination to win the war. Although certain decision-making authorities could be identified as the responsible parties, Ford's article certainly set the scene for a thoroughgoing analysis of why it is that persons in authority were able to make arguments favoring attacks on civilians with credibility in the societies and for the citizenry they represented. The possibility and plausibility of a certain line of reasoning was dependent on a collective bias toward the moral irreproachability of the Allies' cause and the moral (not only military)) necessity of whatever would produce victory. Yet analysis of the social setting of uses of double effect was only hinted at and not really accomplished by the proportionalist critique.

The "analogy" of proportionate reason needs to expand beyond the three alternatives for individual agents that McCormick presents. The Christian and/or human decisions of agents to act or refrain from acting imply a much bigger picture. This is the broader and more complete "common" good (or distorted common good, or common evil) that

establishes individuals' commitments and makes
their reasoning persuasive. This common good is
a network of institutional and structural relationships, along with their guiding narratives, symbols
of meaning, and derivative practices. This inclusive
ethos and set of social relations is defined ideally as
"the common good." But, as proportionalists begin
to suggest, it more often in real life constitutes an
incomplete and distorted good, to which we must
apply a hermeneutic of structural (and not only individual) sin. And let us not forget that institutional
structures are just as important as individual moral
character in helping us do good. It is through social
institutions and networks that we touch the good of
distant others. Institutional pathways of responsibility and accountability are especially crucial for what
recent popes have termed "the universal common
good."

   In an essay five years after *Ambiguity in Moral
Choice*, McCormick reasserts that "proportionate
reasoning represents above all a structure of moral
reasoning" that is "teleological in character."[23] By
this he means that it is forward moving and expan-
sionist. It bears within itself an impetus to social
ethics. In this later essay, McCormick uses illustra-
tions that more readily evoke a social context, than
the examples of *Ambiguity in Moral Choice* (e.g., the
drowning swimmer). McCormick specifically alludes
to the depredations of World War II and Vietnam.
He asks rhetorically, "Is anyone willing to assert

confidently that there is no connection between
Nagasaki-Hiroshima and the senseless slaughters
that occurred in South Vietnam?"[24] McCormick
does not at this point turn to an analysis of structural
sin, and the ethics of collective behavior, both of
which had already been on the table for some time
in Protestant ethics, especially through the writings
of the theologians of the social gospel[25] and of
Reinhold Niebuhr.[26] In Catholic ethics, they were
just beginning to emerge as political and liberation
theology.[27]

As a "moral theologian" (not in those days to
be conflated with a social ethicist), McCormick
strove mightily to demonstrate that something in
certain acts themselves, including acts of war, while
seemingly only acting against a "premoral good"
like physical life, and hence in theory justifiable
by proportionate reason, actually harm some other
important good in the association of basic goods that
make up human flourishing, and so can be prohibited across the boards. In other words, he argues, even
in the isolated act of an individual agent or body, a
social injustice is committed that leads unavoidably
to further acts of injustice in the future. "That is
why," McCormick believes, "the Christian judges
attacks upon noncombatants as disproportionate."
Here, I believe, the reasoning becomes contorted
or forced, and not ultimately compelling. "In such
an attack—even though more lives might be saved
than trying to grind the war to a halt by conven-

tional methods—liberty is at stake [the liberty of the aggressor to desist] and to undermine it is to turn against the basic good of life itself. For these goods are...associated."[28] Or again, the killing of noncombatants in warfare "is disproportionate to the good being sought because it undermines through the association of basic goods the very good of life."[29] In such acts, "wrongfulness must be attributed to a lack of proportion."[30]

Beside the fact that the argument about not violating the liberty of the adversary to cease aggression would seem to preclude any act of war or coercion, the maneuver of trying to attach all the social causes and consequences of unjust warfare to specific moral decisions considered in themselves seems highly unpersuasive. While it is commendable to regard such decisions with high moral seriousness, and to hold their perpetrators individually and personally accountable, the analogical thrust of proportionate reasoning suggests a broadening of the moral scope to include a straightforwardly structural analysis. Even if the killing of an innocent person in warfare in some rare and extreme case *cannot* be ruled out in principle in the nature of the case, public justification and general tolerance of such a practice would be unwise. It would run the danger of dehumanizing both perpetrators and victims, and of further underwriting the cruelty and disrespect for human beings that already motivates the preponderance of world affairs. The murder of noncombatants also exemplifies and perpetuates the huge inequalities of power that already exist between warring governments and the populations within which their savagery is carried out, as well as the disproportionate power and lust for dominance that propel war's engines and place the defeated in the victor's hands. The moral-theological mindset of double effect, even in revised "proportionalist" form, just cannot contain this necessary analytic trajectory.

I do not believe that any one revisionist analysis of double effect in light of proportionate reason has ever carried the day. The same is true of the defenders of the "traditional" position who attempt to rebut the critics. In his Marquette lecture, for example, William May expresses an understandable concern about the dangers of creeping consequentialism and of arbitrary judgments, and strives to maintain absolute respect for inviolable moral values such as life, health, truth, beauty and friendship.[31] However, he asserts rather than demonstrates that all such goods are equal and absolute (would one never sacrifice beauty for health, health for life?), and he misrepresents what it is that the "proportionalists" actually maintain. Says he, "they even claim that a person *can* at times freely choose to do what he or she believes to be gravely immoral…and still remain, in the core of his or her being, a morally good person."[32] Surely all parties to this debate agree both that choosing something one knows to be immoral is a sin, and that otherwise good people can sin gravely and still return to a better path.

Most problematically, however, the model of analysis May uses is fixed indefatigably on an individual agent whose personal freedom knows few bounds. May thinks "the truth of moral absolutes" can and does depend on "the significance of human acts as free, self-determining choices."[33] "The truth, in short, is that we determine our selves, our being as moral persons, in and through the actions we freely choose to do each day."[34] While May is certainly right to affirm the human freedom without which responsibility is impossible, I would add that the social encyclicals of recent popes deplore the consumerism, materialism, and militarism of societies like ours precisely because they have such a deforming effect on human identity, consciousness and "freedom."

In sum, double effect thinking and proportionalism suffer from a common shortcoming. They take principles and rules that have evolved as short-hand, experience-based safeguards against biased thinking and action, and turn these prudential maxims into logically necessary and practically absolute characteristics of individual moral behavior. As scholars of casuistry have already shown,[35] principles like double effect were refined, eclectically and over centuries, precisely to guide analogical thinking that compared present situations to dilemmas that had been satisfactorily resolved in the past.

In the era of globalization particularly, the situations that concern bioethicists cannot be studied and resolved on the basis of a model directed to the consideration of the nature and structure of acts alone. Even an exploration of the contexts of particular agents is not adequate to this task. The "proportionate reason" of the new bioethics must be the universal common good. The obligations, intentions and actions that pertain to the common good must be appreciated and assessed in light of their social, corporate, and institutional character. Human freedom, especially social freedom, is always dragged down by the weight of personal and social sin and the structures that mediate and reinforce sin. Useful here is the proposal with which McCormick concluded *Ambiguity in Moral Choice*: though morality is "objective," the discernment of proportionate reason is inductive, the possibilities of conflict resolution multiple, and judgments often "rationally untidy."[36]

McCormick on Death and Dying

The evolution of proportionate reason toward an ethics of the common good in bioethics can be traced by means of a review of some of McCormick's writings on the subject of death and dying. One of the perennial and central concerns of Catholic "moral theology" has been decision-making in situations where human health and life are at stake. This has been true of moral theology throughout its develop-

ment from medieval confessors' manuals to the late
nineteenth and mid twentieth-century neoscholastic
moral textbooks. For example, Gerald Kelly, S.J.,
who wrote one of the most influential medical ethics
manuals for North American moral theologians of
the last generation,[37] credits the distinction between
ordinary and extraordinary means of life support to
a seventeenth-century Spanish Cardinal, John de
Lugo, relying on predecessors such as Tomas Sanchez
(sixteenth century) and informing interpreters such
as Alphonsus Liguouri (eighteenth century).[38] This
is an old distinction still in use today, and one that
has always had latent social ramifications.[39]

Perhaps McCormick's single best-known piece
on this topic is a short essay on decision-making in
the case of a baby boy who was born with multiple
life-threatening physical abnormalities, and probable
serious mental impairment. Entitled "To Save or Let
Die,"[40] the essay is written against the backdrop of
the principle of double effect and the distinction
between ordinary and extraordinary means of life
support. The social context of the essay was the technological development of neonatal intensive care,
and the resultant need for families and medical teams
to make decisions about whether and when to sustain
the lives of children who faced inevitable eventual
death anyway, or a gravely blighted life. Decisions
to decline or withdraw treatment had come under
fire in some quarters, due to a concern that the end
of life for many infants was being judged accept-

able primarily to avoid burdens to family members or society. At the same time, it seemed to many caregivers that continued life would not always be a blessing to children who come into this world with irremediable physical disabilities, often causing poor prospects for intelligent consciousness as well.

As McCormick saw it, "it is safe to say that public discussion of such controversial issues will quickly collapse into slogans such as 'There is no such thing as a life not worth saving,' or 'Who is the physician to play God?'" On the other side, "'death with dignity' translates for many into a death that is fast, clean, painless."[41] McCormick's article attempts to surface the values involved, subject them to scrutiny, and provide a hermeneutic of decision-making that is consistent with Catholic teaching and that makes medical and moral common sense.

Moving toward his own proposal, McCormick mentions an analysis by James Gustafson of a decision to withhold treatment from a baby that had been born with Down Syndrome at Johns Hopkins hospital.[42] McCormick praises Gustafson for having in a nondogmatic way criticized decision-makers who had subordinated the good of an infant to the needs and wishes of parents. The child, after all, had a chance at a happy and even constructive life, even if not a "normal" one. Yet the parents felt themselves unable to shoulder the strain of raising a mentally disabled child. What Gustafson did not provide was an overarching value or set of values that could be definitive in such cases, nor a criterion or set of criteria that could be applied to similar cases in the future.

McCormick attempts to supply these by drawing on the Catholic tradition on the positive meaning of life, and on the distinction between ordinary and extraordinary means of life support. These resources allow McCormick to attend to the contexts of the decision and of the infant's life prospects, and to address, at least implicitly, the problems of structural or institutionalized bias that inhere in the North American medical system. These include a preference for highly technological medical care, a rather individualistic practice of "autonomous" decision-making, and a social predisposition to value highly productive human beings and to regard the mentally impaired as incapable of truly "meaningful" life. McCormick agrees that "quality of life" judgments are necessary, but he insists that the judgment of quality be made from the perspective of the disabled individual himself or herself. Quality must not be equated simplistically with a life free of suffering or with the sorts of enjoyments or accomplishments that are ordinarily regarded as "normal."

The guiding value or good in a human life, McCormick argues, is the psycho-spiritual good of union with God, manifest in this life largely through relationship with and love of other persons. McCormick cites an address of Pope Pius XII, in which he alludes to a "higher more important spiritual good," in service of which physical life is given.[43] This same address also invokes the difference between ordinary and extraordinary means of life support:

> This duty [of preserving life] that one has toward himself, toward God, toward the human community, and in most cases toward certain determined persons, derives from well ordered charity, from submission to the Creator, from social justice and even from strict justice, as well as from devotion toward one's family.
>
> But normally one is held to use only ordinary means—according to circumstances of persons, places, times, and culture—that is to say, means that do not involve any grave burden for oneself or another. A more strict obligation would be too burdensome for most men and would render the attainment of the higher, more important good too difficult. Life, health, all temporal activities, are in fact subordinated to spiritual ends.[44]

We may note here that the principle of double effect and the distinction between ordinary and extraordinary means converge in the fact that the latter distinction is applied in order to avoid the causation of death by direct killing (mercy-killing or euthanasia). The tradition categorizes direct killing of an "innocent" person as an "intrinsically evil act," even if that death is requested by the person or is arguably for the person's own good. Euthanasia is ruled out, even in cases of dire suffering. However, employing

the principle of double effect, one might see relief of
suffering as a good effect and death as a tolerated bad
one, if death were brought about "indirectly," and
were not the outcome desired in itself. Therefore it
is permissible, according to this principle, to refuse
some treatments even if death results, or to use measures to relieve pain that will cause death to come
about faster.[45] Although direct killing is forbidden,
indirect killing by refusing "extraordinary means" is
permissible; but when is it permissible?

Taking into consideration the work of traditional
moralists such as Gerald Kelly, McCormick offers
that quality of life is a valid consideration in decisions whether or not to employ medical treatment.
Such a judgment should refer to the interests of
the ill person himself or herself, above all but may
take into account the relationship between the life
and treatment of that individual and the interests
and needs of others who will be affected by a decision.[46] "Grave hardship" either for oneself or others
could be enough to place a treatment in the nonobligatory or "extraordinary" category. For example,
"older moralists" thought the hardship of moving
to another climate or country was enough to make
a treatment extraordinary, as would the prospect of
life in a severely mutilated state, or the necessity to
undergo surgery without anesthesia. "Similarly, if the
financial cost of life-preserving care was crushing,
that is, if it would create grave hardships for oneself

or one's family, it was considered extraordinary and nonobligatory."[47]

The aspect of this tradition that McCormick develops is the implication that a life preserved in a state of mental impairment or suffering that would drastically interfere with one's ability to recognize and return the love of other persons is a life not worth preserving to the individual living it. Human relationships are the most important part of life, the part that leads us ultimately into relationship with God. "This is not a question about the inherent value of the individual. It is a question about whether this worldly existence will offer such a valued individual any hope of sharing those values for which physical life is the fundamental condition. Is not the only alternative an attitude that supports mere physical life as long as possible with every means?"[48] McCormick, with the help of the tradition on ordinary and extraordinary means of life support, is able to answer this question by saying that respect for the value of an individual can be consistent with removing or declining life-supporting treatment, and allowing death to ensue. This is so if and when treatment is not proportionate to the good of the person, understood as capacity for relationship with other persons and God.

Having begun "To Save or Let Die" with the case of a baby in such disastrous physical condition that survival is unlikely and "quality of life" extremely low by just about any measure, McCormick is able

to illustrate and apply his "relational potential" criterion in a relatively trouble-free and decisive way.
However, this particular case allows him, once again,
to narrow the focus of analysis to the relationships
life does or does not hold for one infant. Subsequent
intra-Catholic debates about withholding or with-
drawing treatment, for example artificial nutrition
and hydration,[49] have for the most part adhered to a
similar focus. In order to avoid the reality or accusa-
tion of utilitarianism, Catholic thinkers have argued
that their proposed solutions to these difficult cases,
whether for or against foregoing different types of
treatment, are based primarily on the welfare of an
individual patient, and whether or not a decision
serves that good. For instance, McCormick himself,
in arguing for the removal of feeding tubes from
comatose patients, keeps the individual patient at
the center of attention when he concludes that a
treatment may be omitted "if it is useless or futile,
or if it imposes burdens that outweigh the benefits."
The "true heart" of the issue, he believes, is whether
"such a life" is "a value to the one in such a state," and
he believes (in accord, he argues, with the Vatican's
Declaration on Euthanasia) that it is not.[50]

The decision-making process becomes a good
deal murkier if it is not so clear or not clear at all
that the life preserved will be unduly burdensome
"to the patient," but more clear that it will be a
burden, especially an undue burden, to others (as in
the Down Syndrome case considered by Gustafson).

McCormick would undoubtedly say that, in such a case, the infant has a life worth living and should be sustained. However, once social considerations have been introduced, they are not so easily disposed of. In the Johns Hopkins case, as presented by Gustafson, the parents in question at least had access to resources and might have come though counseling and support to envision a way in which they could accept the disabled child into their family. Circumstances might be radically other.

We have all heard accounts of desperate refugee mothers who have smothered their wailing infants so that a fleeing party not be detected and massacred by pursuers. Who among us has had the moral nerve to condemn such women, or to accuse them of holding the lives of their babies of little account, when confronted with a choice between the death of one or the death of all? What about mothers in situations of desperate poverty or famine, who have systematically deprived one or more children of nourishment, so that their siblings might retain a tenuous grasp on life? A doctor from the Philippines writes that AIDS patients in her country, with its strong ethos of individual commitment to family welfare, frequently forego drug treatment for their disease, "so that whatever resources are left maybe used by their family and loved ones for a better future."[51] Traditional authors, including Pius XII, provocatively and all too briefly mention cost and burden to family members and communities as considerations that

can make treatments "extraordinary." They never
fine-tune the significance of this possibility for the
worth and rights of the individual, nor address the
morality of the conditions that make such choices
necessary, nor elaborate on how the common good
can or cannot comprehend the goods of all individual
parties to conflict cases.

To complicate the problem further, consider the
fact that family and community resources affect the
quality of life prospects of ill individuals themselves,
even if all decision-makers are committed to providing whatever care is available. How greatly dependent
is the assessment of "burden to the patient" on the
availability to that patient and his or her care-givers
of social and medical support systems? Different
supports are accessible if one lives within range of
a major medical center in a wealthy industrialized
country, and if one has health insurance, than if
one does not. What if parents in a Brazilian *favela*,
a surviving oldest sibling in an African village rav-
aged by AIDS, or an undocumented immigrant
family in the U.S. claim that they are "too poor" or
"too overburdened" to provide basic care for, much
less medical treatment for, a precarious newborn or
a comatose elder? Is it really adequate to approach
their situations via the principles of double effect
and extraordinary means as applied to the actions
they, specifically, are about to undertake? For one
thing, family members threatened with death in such
situations may indeed have little or no prospect for

a life in meaningful, conscious relationship to God and others, not because innate personal characteristics preclude it, but because the social conditions of life for that person simply deny and negate his or her flourishing. For another, the need to stretch resources in a situation where some must inevitably die of deprivation means that no one individual can be the sole focus of decision.

Although "in theory," parents and families should sustain all lives where minimum conditions of life and consciousness are present, and should never even indirectly sacrifice the potentially worthwhile life of an afflicted individual for the well-being of others, realities may be more ambiguous "in practice." The contextuality of choices and acts includes social structures and institutions that provide conditions for the flourishing of some lives and the grievous deprivation of others. "Proportionate reason" analogously understood propels our attention onward to the common goods and bads of the communal, national, and global social structures that define local contexts of decision-making and construct the "freedom" of agents as the ability to select among what may be very limited and dehumanizing alternatives.

The Common Good and Bioethics

The "dignity of the person" and "the common good" have always been correlative concepts in Catholic social thought. John S. Boswell calls "person" and "common good" the "gateway concepts" of Catholic social teaching. [52] The welfare of all individual persons is contingent upon the interdependent social relations that constitute the common good. Yet the common good is a value in its own right, as more than the aggregate of the individuals participating in it. As we have seen, the common good, and not only individual goods, is an increasingly influential parameter of ethical decisions and practices in the spheres of health and health care.

In the past, little attention was paid to the social and economic effects on communal health care resources of decisions that, considered in isolation, had been deemed morally in accord with Church teaching and the natural law. In Catholic medical ethics, the area that received the highest degree of "contextual" analysis was the morality of decisions about life-prolonging treatment. Yet even though patients were permitted to consider socially contingent factors like spiritual welfare, expense, and burden on family members, it was still the patient-focused situation that governed the analysis. The question of social relations was addressed from the patient's perspective only, not within any larger view of how an individual and his or her needs and interests might fit into or impinge upon the needs of a larger community or of wider individual claims on resources.[53] This assertion should be qualified by adding that the condemnation of direct euthanasia or mercy-killing was very much influenced by consideration of broader social effects. Still, the ultimate concern was a social climate that risked the right to life of vulnerable *individuals*. Institutional analysis in its own right was not a significant part of the picture in official Catholic teaching until the 1990's.[54]

For instance, the 1975 edition of the *Ethical and Religious Directives for Catholic Health Facilities* issued by the U.S. Bishops included in its opening paragraph the declaration that health care providers witness to Christ "by humble service to humanity and especially to the poor."[55] The document does not illuminate the social or public responsibility that might exist in regard to the needs of the poor, nor does it detail the specifics of such service as incumbent on individual providers. The topic areas of most concern, reproductive decisions and end-of-life care, are discussed without reference to social contexts such as gender equality or access to life-prolonging resources. In no way do the 1975 *Directives* overtly challenge the organization of health care so that access is limited to those with financial resources. Its main focus is the dignity and welfare of the individual person, considered in "his" totality and in light of the integrity of "his" bodily functions. The dignity of the person is invoked to preclude any violations of Catholic teaching about the morality of individual acts. However, the dignity of the person is not linked to the morality of institutions that distribute health care unequally, thus predetermining the options that are open to individual choice.

In contrast, the 2001 edition of the *Directives* contains a substantial introductory section on "the social responsibility of Catholic health care services." The commitment of Catholic health care both to human dignity and to the common good is affirmed. The "biblical mandate to care for the poor" should be expressed "in concrete action at all levels of Catholic health care," including work to ensure that the health care delivery system is accountable to the needs of the poor and uninsured. "Responsible stewardship" of health resources is held up as an obligation to seek equitable care and to promote "the good health of all in the community," in dialogue with people from all levels of society in accordance with the principle of subsidiarity.[56]

A social perspective now informs questions that were once simply treated under the rubric of intrinsically evil or permissible individual acts. Rather than limiting itself to a blunt condemnation of direct abortion, the new *Directives* stipulates that

> The church's defense of life encompasses the unborn and the care of women and their children during and after pregnancy. The Church's commitment to life is seen in its willingness to collaborate with others to alleviate the causes of the high infant mortality rate and to provide adequate health care to mothers and their children before and after birth.[57]

In the context of access to health care and the right to health care decision-making, the *Directives* states, "The inherent dignity of the human person must be respected and protected regardless of the nature of the person's health problem or social status. The respect for human dignity extends to all persons who are served by Catholic health care."[58]

Pope John Paul II takes this critical vision, of the link between human dignity and access to health care via just institutions, to the level of the universal common good. He warned in 2003 that there is a

> very serious and unacceptable gap that separates the developing world from the developed in terms of the capacity to develop biomedical research for the benefit of health care assistance and to assist peoples afflicted by chronic poverty and dire epidemics....It is essential to realize that to leave these peoples without the resources of science and culture means to condemn them to poverty, financial exploitation and the lack of health care structures, and also to commit an injustice and fuel a long-term threat for the globalized world.[59]

At both the national and the global levels, health care is a collective responsibility, and it extends to provision of the conditions of health that are as basic as food, clean water, shelter, and immunity from sexual coercion. It also includes preventive medicine, emergency care, treatment for chronic illness, accom-

modation for disabilities, and appropriate medical
support in old age and in the dying process.

The last decade has seen a mounting debate over
health care reform in the United States. Though
hardly resolved, the injustice of excluding forty million people from access to the health care system in
the wealthiest country in the world has now become
a prominent feature of the national political agenda.
Philip Keane concludes that "access to a reasonable
level of health care remains a clear obligation of
distributive justice, an inviolable human right, and
a basic requirement of the common good." The
individual's right to health care is "part of an integrated continuum with the greater good of society,"
since individual rights are part of the calling of all
to social responsibility.[60]

Clarke and David Cochran emphasize that "discrimination, denial of care, and neglect of essential
needs injure community. How can we claim to
serve the common good, when we deny essential
healthcare to millions?"[61] The Cochrans note that
healthcare research and development result in more
technology, which is driven into U.S. healthcare by
the market as much as by need. This has implications
for stewardship of resources and their just distribution. The market depends on an individualistic
rather than on a social perspective, treats health as a
commodity rather than as a basic need, and deprives
those without financial assets of health care while
encouraging the development of biomedical inno-

vations that can be sold to the privileged few. The Church, its members, its health care institutions, and Catholic bioethics must respond by "institutional presence, leadership and witness, and public policy advocacy."[62] Reform of the health care system requires the cooperative action of state and federal governments and legislation, civil society and local organizations, and the individual commitment of every citizen and voter. The Catholic Church is an organization that can respond along all these social and institutional axes, showing individuals where their responsibilities lie, and encouraging social participation for change.

This multifaceted process can be endorsed on the basis of a staple of the encyclicals, the "principle of subsidiarity," especially if it is interpreted in a more sophisticated way to meet the challenges of globalization and of interdependence among peoples and nations. The principle of subsidiarity entered Catholic social teaching with Pius XI's *Quadragesimo Anno* (1930). It can be interpreted to affirm cooperative responsibility for the common good between smaller, more local units of society and larger, more comprehensive associations and authorities, such as the federal government.[63] Although big government should not take over what local government and civil society can accomplish, a higher authority intervention is sometimes required to right imbalances in local preferences and practices.

Andrew Lustig applies Catholic teaching on ownership of private property to bioethics in this regard.
From the first of the modern papal social encyclicals,
Leo XIII's *Rerum Novarm* (1891), onward private
property has been viewed as a nonabsolute good, to
which individuals or groups have a right only insofar
as their ownership interferes neither with the rights
of other individuals nor with the common good.
Insofar as they pertain to material well-being, health
care resources can be included under the rubric of
private property. Therefore individual consumers do
not have a right to utilize disproportionate resources,
even if they can pay for them, if their use interferes
with the access of others who lack a decent minimum
of care. The federal government has an obligation
to reallocate resources by establishing different patterns of access, if the market-based system now in
place in the U.S. works to the disadvantage of the
least well-off.[64]

When we move to the level of global health
resources, however, the standard "local to national"
understanding of subsidiarity starts to break down.
First of all, there is no one global government with
the power, over and above the consent of individual
nations, to reallocate resources internationally.
Nevertheless, and more positively for the prospects
of health care justice, it seems that reallocation can
and does occur, at least to some degree, through the
interaction of a variety of agents at lower levels. These
include governmental and nongovernmental organi-

zations, advocacy networks, and political coalitions, as well as "world" organizations such as the United Nations and World Health Organization. These sites of agency and change are not simply located on a two-way spectrum from "smaller" to "bigger." They arise both horizontally and vertically, in many shifting constellations of action and reaction, in which group membership often overlaps.

One example of such action for change is the struggle of poor countries to obtain AIDS drugs, occurring over the past three years or so. The need of the poor for cheaper or free versions of patented AIDS drugs became much more visible internationally as a result of a dispute between the government of South Africa and major pharmaceutical companies. The point in contention was World Trade Organization regulations prohibiting the manufacture and sale of generic AIDS drugs in competition with patents held by multinational corporations. Eventually, as a result of pressure from a number of sources, including Oxfam, Doctors without Borders, and the UN, as well as AIDS activists, WTO rules were adjusted. Countries in need (led by Brazil) began to manufacture and distribute generics, and an international "Global Fund to Fight AIDS, Malaria and TB," based in Geneva, was established in 2003 to elicit and distribute donations to address the crisis.[65] Though the response is as yet far from adequate to the need, it demonstrates that multi-leveled activism and accountability can bring results.

It also shows that the neatly hierarchical ordering of concentric circles of society that is suggested by the traditional categories of Catholic social teaching does not describe the realities of the common good at the global level. "Subsidiarity" can be redefined to meet this new situation if it is expanded horizontally, recognizing and affirming the "authority" over society and politics that can be exercised through the participatory collaboration of a variety of morally committed actors in the national, international, and transnational spheres.

Global Health Needs and the Common Good
According to the WHO's *World Health Report 2003*,[66] HIV/AIDS has cut life expectancy by as much as twenty years for many millions of people in sub-Saharan Africa, with only 5% of those requiring antiretroviral treatment actually receiving it. In developing countries, communicable diseases still represent seven out the ten major causes of child deaths. In Africa, malaria is the number one killer of children under five. The leading causes of death for adults, in addition to AIDS in Africa, are respiratory infections, diarrhea, and malaria. Some 500 million people in Africa, Asia, and Latin America are infected by malaria each year. Annual deaths worldwide from malaria are conservatively estimated at more than 1.2 million, ninety percent of them in Africa. The risk for women dying in childbirth is 250 times greater for women in poor countries than in rich ones,

with more than 500, 000 women a year dying from complications of pregnancy. In sub-Saharan Africa, AIDS orphans already number around 12 million, and is estimated to reach 20 million by 2010.[67]

Though it is obvious that poor people, especially in poor countries, will suffer and die from lack of access to health care, Norman Daniels and co-authors have detailed the links between a variety of forms of participation in the common good and their impact on health. They observe that even in countries that offer the poor access to health services, those services will be underutilized, and health will be worse, among the poor. Both access and utilization are tied to other social indicators of status and self-respect, such as education, gender equality, and a positive work environment.[68] Veena Das uses examples of states in India to make the complementary point that good and poor government correlates with equal and unequal health resource distribution (such as immunization), partly because the poor have little representation in nondemocratic, authoritarian or bureaucratic governments. Moreover, government health programs may be met with "relative apathy" in the face of much more urgent survival needs, or in the face of barriers to access like lack of education as to the purpose and potency of medicines, transportation, or permission from family or village authorities to take advantage of the resources offered.[69] Health and health care, as basic conditions of human flourishing, exemplify the interdependence of all aspects of participation in the common good of society. Health care cannot be addressed as a social justice concern without also addressing multiple relationships in the entire social fabric of which health is a part.

The cultural and religious worldviews of distinct communities can also influence the way that health and life are integrated into the common good, as well as the types of institutions and of social participation though which persons enjoy health, cope with illness, and define human well-being in general. Although many basic elements of human needs and welfare remain the same among cultures, cultural differences are reflected in the way health and illness, medicine, and death and suffering are interpreted and confronted. Unfortunately from the standpoint of other cultures, Western market economics, hi-tech medicine, and individual autonomy-centered bioethics have managed to force their influence around the globe.[70]

In African and Asian societies, the community is much more clearly prior to the individual than it is in the U.S., and decisions about how to distribute common resources among family members or how to deal with illness, are family-centered, not gauged by individual needs. Often it is the family, or elders and authorities within the family, who make decisions regarding the needs of individuals. Describing the situation in the Philippines, Angeles Tan Alora and Josephine Lumitao describe the primary moral agent in health issues as "the familial community."

> The family is considered to be the social unit of greatest value in the Filipino culture. The family is the core of all social and economic activity. It provides emotional security, economic support, and a deep sense of belonging…. Given this strong family ethos, the primary locus of assessment of the good is not the individual but the family. Maintenance of harmony within the family and among peers takes precedence over other concerns for social justice or honesty, which from this perspective appear to be anonymous formal principles that are disengaged from concrete moral life…. As a consequence, Western ideals of individualism and self-reliance have little purchase in the Filipino culture.[71]

This ethos has a decisive effect is decision-making about treatment in times of serious or terminal illness, including the use of life-prolonging measures. Lumitao notes that the cost of health care in the Philippines is borne almost entirely by the family. She adds, "such high costs qualify most treatment for dying patients as extraordinary. Justification for withdrawal of treatment on financial grounds is not difficult."[72] She gives the example of a seventeen year old boy who was injured in a car accident, and consequently was paralyzed from the neck down. He could survive with mental faculties intact, but only with the permanent use of a ventilator. When his family was advised of this prognosis, the young man "looked sad," but after a few days asked for the ventilator to be removed. He had six younger siblings, and the hospital bills were mounting far beyond the modest means of his family.[73] Yet, according to Lumitao, Filipinos rarely entertain thoughts of euthanasia, because close family support, acceptance of suffering, and religious trust in eternal life create an ethos where that is a culturally inconceivable option.[74]

This case exemplifies a number of discrepancies between bioethics in the U.S. and in the developing world, even in the limited context of Catholic teaching and principles. First of all, while the person and community are seen as interdependent in Catholic thought generally, thinkers such as McCormick and William May tend to assume the availability of resources, and focus on the welfare of the individual patient. Secondly, they assume that the decision-maker is the patient himself or herself, or a substitute or proxy whose duty it is to represent the patient's interests. Thirdly, they rarely if ever develop the possibility that a means could become "extraordinary" by virtue of a family's inability to pay, if that means could allow the patient to live a meaningful life. Yet such conflicts are acknowledged in magisterial and theological writings. Finally, first world authors should and would identify the fact that many people among the less wealthy classes in less wealthy countries are excluded from access to treatments as a form of social injustice. But they avoid the fact that actual, *de facto* existence in circumstances of injustice might change the nature of the objectively right moral act. They fail to recognize that such circumstances might create real moral conflict, not just apparent conflicts, or conflicting premoral goods. This occurs when none of the choices available are the one or ones that theories of double effect, extraordinary means, human dignity and rights, common good, etc., would identify as ideal or commendable. Sometimes the dignity of the person and the common good cannot be kept in balance.

Theologians and bioethicists in the U.S. are developing programs and analyses to counteract the bias toward high technology end-of-life care, primarily to provide a more humane context for the end of life, and partly in view of more efficient and just use of resources. Hospice care and palliative care, either in the hospital or in another context, are increasingly extolled as important and preferable alternatives, medically, morally and spiritually.[75] Yet we rarely contemplate the possibility that "ordinary" life-prolonging measures in the U.S. context might very well become "extraordinary" if global health needs were taken into account, and that what bests serves "the higher more important good" for a given individual would have to be sacrificed for the good of the community. North Americans, at least in "mainstream," middle class culture, are rarely forced to envision

the possibility that expensive measures that would
be truly beneficial to themselves or their loved ones
would be unavailable in a just world, because such
benefits would have to be eliminated from the global
health system for all to have basic preventive care and
therapies for curable diseases. An important voice in
this regard is Daniel Callahan, who has frequently
criticized the American avoidance of the reality of
aging and death, obsession with intensive end-of-life
care, and wasteful, selfish use of health care resources.
Callahan has also suggested that some lines need to
be drawn on what "we" have a right to use, even if
it is useful to us. His focus has been on cost-cutting
and redistribution within the U.S. however.[76]

Person and Common Good:
Co-dependence and Conflict

In theory, the two concepts of personal dignity
and common good cannot be separated. They are
interdependent and mutually reinforcing. Major
Catholic thinkers, preeminently Jacques Maritain,
have shown, at least in principle, that, due to the
social nature of the person, neither society nor person
can exist without the other; neither can be sacrificed.
Their interdependence, recognized and implemented
as the moral framework of human life, is the very
meaning of the common good. The common good is
"the good human life of the multitude, of a multitude
of persons; it is their communion in good living. It is
therefore common to both the whole and the parts

into which it flows back and which, in turn, must benefit from it."[77]

The examples above have illustrated, however, that the convergence of common and individual needs cannot always be presupposed at the ground level. The traditional Catholic focus on the inviolability of individual rights and responsibilities can be unrealistic and intransigent in light of the conflicts of real life. Nevertheless, the insistence that "the dignity of the person" is co-originate with and just as important as the common good is important as a sort of moral sign-post. It is a form of practical moral commitment to resist rather than capitulate to sinful social forces that oppress persons. In contrast, utilitarianism — resisted by both traditionalist and revisionist Catholic thinkers — can be seen, not so much as a type of disregard for the worth of individuals, as a form of resignation to the fact that the "real world" does not allow even equally regarded individuals to be equally the objects of our beneficence. Thus the most moral policy is to seek at least the greatest good for the greatest number possible.

By keeping together the common good and the dignity of the person, Catholic moral thinking insists that the conflicts and ambiguities of life be resolved within the perennial tension of active respect for both. The stress on the individual person represents resistance to evil and a transformative agenda against the "powers" that force ambiguous choices; the stress on the *common good* acknowledges that individuals are converted and their good served only within the structures and practices within which they come into being and define themselves, and that no individual rights supersede social responsibility.

In practical decisions and policies, however, the tension between justice as equal respect, and as beneficence or utility, has still not disappeared. Virtually any case of scarce medical resources can illustrate this point. It is particularly acute in the case of those health benefits that are in the nature of the case impossible to share around equally among a large number of people (organs for transplant), or whose efficacy will be lost if they are (AIDS medications). A few months ago I saw a photograph in the New York Times of a man with AIDS and his young daughter, also afflicted by the disease.[78] Able to scrounge enough money for only one regimen of AIDS drugs, the man was taking them himself, on the rationale that his support was needed by the whole family. The ten-year-old daughter received none. One could argue both that the little girl was being treated with less respect than the man, and that the welfare of the family was best served by the decision he had made. One could also say that the father's action, considered in itself, could be justified by the principles of double effect and of extraordinary means. He was only "indirectly" killing his daughter, and the cost of the treatment for her would place an "extraordinary" burden on the family, which would then stand to lose its main provider.

This assessment may be true as far as it goes, but it hardly seems adequate. Surely the point of the story was to highlight the moral necessity for privileged readers of the *New York Times* to take action in making AIDS drugs available and affordable in Zambia, where the family lived, and in similar places worldwide. The proper focus if moral analysis of the story is institutional and social. To insist on the "equal dignity" of the daughter is not in the end a way of saying that the father's decision according to the principle of utility was immoral, or that he could and should have chosen in another way that protected his daughter and his family equally. (It is, though, a way of raising the possibility that a social bias against the equal worth of women and girls could have influenced his decision.) Insisting on the daughter's dignity as a person, despite the fact that her good was concretely incompatible with that of other family members, is ultimately a way of holding other persons, groups, segments of society, nations, and the international community to account because the father's choice was "forced." It is a way of surfacing the likelihood that the wealthy nations' concern about this little girl's fate is biased because she is black, poor, and lives in Africa.

John Boswell has suggested that the distinctive character of Catholic social thought lies in the fact that justice is always linked with subsidiarity and solidarity, with solidarity "at the peak."[79] Solidarity has been defined by John Paul II as "the moral and social attitude" or "virtue" that corresponds to the recognition of interdependence ("economic, cultural, political and religious") as a "moral category." Solidarity is "a *firm and persevering determination* to commit oneself to the *common good*."[80] The pope also believes that solidarity informed by faith is able to conquer "'structures of sin.'" It represents "a *diametrically opposed attitude*" that seeks the neighbor's good, especially through service instead of exploitation and the oppression of others to one's own advantage. Perhaps most importantly for the revised understanding of subsidiarity as much more multidimensional that previously recognized, solidarity is growing positively among the poor themselves. John Paul II gives affirmation to the fact that they "*support one another*" and engage in "*public demonstrations* on the social scene" in order to assert their own needs and rights to the "public authorities."[81]

In Boswell's view, solidarity is a broader social analogue to love, and includes "relationships of community, sociability, conviviality, civility, *fraternité*, civic friendship, social consciousness, public spirit." It can arise in interpersonal relations, inter-group relations, and even "supra-national spheres." Boswell uses the phrase "complex solidarity."[82] Informed by solidarity, subsidiarity represents power-sharing. "Power is to be diffused, spreading out both vertically (from citizen, through locality or region, to nation state, and supranationally), and horizontally (in terms of a plurality of political, cultural and economic forms)."[83]

Likewise informed by solidarity, justice is transformed. Absolute equality, in the sense of equal respect for the dignity of each human being, may be utopian. Yet justice demands at least "a less unequal division of resources, a calling to account of the rich and powerful, a raising-up of the poor." Justice becomes more urgent in light of solidarity; it also expands beyond resource distribution to include the full participation of those who have been marginalized. "Their self-organisation, representation and participation are also critical."[84] Two urgent social causes Boswell thus identifies are devolution of political power and radical redistribution to fight poverty.[85] Boswell understands that innovative public forums and institutions are needed to give the various stakeholders in the common good effective voice and vote, and that these must develop interactively with different contexts and trends.[86] The reality is, in fact, that these forums and institutions are already developing "from below" and "from the middle," pressuring and prompting policy changes, rather than following policies authorized "from above." Perhaps there is no way to rule out or resolve in principle all clashes of goods like those that happened in the Filipino and Zambian families I described. However, solidarity, power-sharing and justice as the participation of all stakeholders in decisions would reduce the incidence of such situations and the likelihood that they are resolved to the detriment of the most vulnerable persons.

Implications for Proportionalism

The identification of agency in bioethics as both personal and social, as fully contextual, and as inhering in complex, collective, and interactive modes of solidaristic participation in the common good helps to address some of the problems or questions that were unresolved by proportionalism. Two types of "ambiguity" were identified by Richard McCormick, as he probed the role of proportionate reason in the application of the principle of double effect. The first of these was ambiguity in the *knowledge* of objective good, or of the objectively right moral act. The second was the inevitability in the real world of *conflicts* between the goods of individuals and the goods of the communities of which they are a part.

The ambiguity of *knowledge* of the good derives from the finitude of human perspective and reasoning, and the fact that finite human reasoning is made even more unreliable by the bias of sin. The function of the principle of double effect is to set limits on the use of proportionate reason, precisely to avoid the distortions that limited perspective and self-interest might introduce into decisions about sexuality, causing death, and even warfare. Recently, authors from Africa and Asia have eloquently named the distortions that can affect whole cultures, when their own cultural perspectives are assumed to be final and comprehensive, and when self-interest guides discernment about what, for example, is fair and just medical resource distribution, investment of research money, or business practice in the marketing and sale of pharmaceutical products. It is evident that moral knowledge is inherently bound up in and dependent on interests, commitments, and practices that identify certain problems as requiring resolution, and certain values as deserving priority in defining the course ahead.

This does not mean that "objectivity" is a meaningless ideal, but rather that knowledge of the morally good and right, can only be approximated by any one seeker, and that participatory, cooperative discernment is essential to understand moral truths. As Maura Ryan states the challenge, "a theological global bioethics" must be "self-critical about the role of families and communities (including faith communities) in creating conditions of unequal and dangerous vulnerability for individuals or groups of individuals, e.g., conditions whereby the world's women are differentially vulnerable to HIV infection and death from untreated AIDS." She suggests that narratives are one useful way of introducing alternative moral frameworks in a cross-cultural bioethics.[87] Narratives, stories, and personal accounts (such as the above cases from the Philippines and Africa) are ways to stimulate the moral imagination, so that a worldview shift begins to occur, opening the hearer to the "reasonableness" of moral warrants and arguments that were incomprehensible or intolerable on the basis of old assumptions and priorities. The acquisition of moral knowledge is an incremental, socially embedded process, especially when trying to address problems of the common good that involve the human dignity of persons from very different cultural and social settings.

This process, even if undertaken collaboratively and in good faith, can never completely eliminate the reality that some *moral conflicts* cannot be resolved in such a way that the good of all persons and the common good are commensurately served, or kept in perfect balance. While one classic way to handle such dilemmas is to seek "the greatest good for the greatest number," the sadly more common way is for every individual or group to promote and fight for his, her, or its own advantage. Greater than the danger of utilitarianism is the danger, I believe, of a libertarian approach to biomedicine and ethics, in which consumers, interest groups, providers, and researchers all do their utmost to grab the biggest piece of the resources, profits, or benefits. Market-based health care, and profit-driven biotechnological research into exotic cures for first-world diseases, offend even more greatly against justice than the idea that global health resources should serve the greatest number of people in the best and most efficient way possible.

A bioethics centered on the dignity of the person and the common good ultimately can accept neither of these solutions (utilitarianism or libertarianism) as fully adequate. I am convinced by McCormick and other critics of traditional moral theology that a deductive application of rules and principles to cases is not adequate either. In fact, the origins of double effect itself are inductive, cumulative, contextual and prudential, far from the way double effect was applied to "hard cases" in the neo-scho-lastic, manualist era. Moral judgment simply cannot escape the need for the virtue of prudence, nor the need to apply practical reason contextually in the dilemmas and quandaries of life. What is different in the emerging bioethics of the common good is that reasoning, judgments and virtues are now more clearly understood to have a social dimension, and to be embodied in and through structures, institutions, and ongoing practices, not only in the "choices" of individual agents.

One outcome of this new appreciation of the social character of agency, judgment, and action, is that moral dilemmas, always arising in social contexts, are seen to be resolvable only in the same contexts. Like Boswell, Francis McHugh names "'the dignity of human nature' and 'the common good'" as the "guid-ing visions for Catholic social thought and action." Yet he grants that this vision must be brought "into connection with the realities of social life and a range of policy questions" through "middle-level thinking," informed by a concern for distributive justice, soli-darity, subsidiarity, and a preferential option for the

poor.[88] The guiding or "proportionate" good in all
situations and decisions must be the common good,
understood as including the dignity of each person.
But the proportionate good that resolves dilemmas
must be understood pluralistically, incorporating the
dignity of the person in different ways and degrees.
As McCormick explained, it may be best in some
instances to sacrifice one's own welfare, while in
others simple justice (permitting each agent to give
a priority to his or her own life) can guide. In still
other situations, the greatest good possible may be
simply to avoid the greater evil.

Now, in view of the intransigence of real moral
conflict, given historical brokenness and the effects
of personal and social sin, we also need to expand
proportionate reason "analogously" in another way.
Sometimes the best solution possible in a given situation, seen in its extenuating social conditions and
ramifications and the pressures they place on decision-makers, is only a solution "analogous" to the
good we truly desire. This happens when families and
societies have to make allocation decisions because
adequate medical care for all is unavailable. Social,
contextual "middle-level thinking" will sometimes
have to search out an imperfect good as a real and
objective, though provisional, good, and choose it as
embodying to the greatest degree concretely possible
justice, solidarity, subsidiarity, and the preferential

option for the poor. Yet its realization may unavoidably upset or tip the balance between the person and the common good. At the end of the day, Gustafson may be right to refrain from delineating absolute rankings of goods, or propounding clear and decisive sets of norms.

AIDS, Bioethics, and the Common Good

The worldwide scourge of AIDS has been outlined above, as though that were needed for an educated audience in the twenty-first century. AIDS is a medical, social, and moral dilemma with which theological bioethicists and the Catholic Church have tried to grapple for over a decade. The literature is immense,[89] and only few key aspects will be treated here. The first point to be made is that when AIDS first came to the attention of Catholic moral theology, its analysis was closely connected to the morality of personal sexual behavior. Specifically, first-world moral theologians and Church teachers perceived AIDS as originating in sexual sin, especially homosexuality (as well as IV drug use). Later, when the global dimensions of the disease became evident, it was and still is associated with promiscuous heterosexual behavior. Hence, the "remedy" for AIDS was perceived to be stricter observance of sexual morality, though Catholic health care ministries also upheld the responsibility to care for those afflicted with AIDS.[90] Gradually, awareness grew that the impact of AIDS on the health of populations around the world is dire.

AIDS began to move out of the category of a sexual problem and into that of a global health problem. It is also a problem of appropriate medical and social responses to suffering and death. Broader social issues began to be examined, including more effective means of preventing transmission (the debate about the use of condoms), the inequities of wealth and power that contribute to the spread of AIDS, the need of resource redistribution to treat all those with AIDS with antiretroviral drugs, and the obligation to care for communities afflicted by AIDS (especially AIDS orphans) as falling on the international community, especially its wealthiest members. AIDS has become a problem of bioethics and the global common good.

One impact that AIDS has had on bioethics has been to force a shift in the way U.S. bioethicists and moral theologians have perceived and approached the ethics of "death and dying." The distinction between ordinary and extraordinary means of life support is not very helpful when the problem is not to decide whether to refuse what is available, but to obtain what is not. The work of theological ethicist Margaret Farley provides an example. Feminist ethicists, both religious and philosophical, have been in the forefront of the movement in bioethics toward social consciousness and advocacy for the deprived.[91] However, like most bioethicists, Farley was originally concerned about whether or not it could be justified for an individual to choose death by direct means, in certain limited circumstances, and for the welfare of the dying person. In order to illustrate the meaning of accepting death as an act of active surrender to God, she chose the example of a young man dying of AIDS in a modern medical center, for whom "no more could be done."[92]

In 2002, Farley developed a "feminist approach to medical ethics and other questions," in which she addressed AIDS as a worldwide problem, one particularly affecting women living in poverty and under cultural norms of vast gender inequality.[93] "Why," she asks, "do women bear a disproportionate share in the burdens of the AIDS pandemic? Without power over their sexual lives, they have little control over occasions of infection….If educated women are at risk, the vulnerability of women increases exponentially when they live in small villages and rural areas without access to medical education."[94] Calling on the Christian virtues of compassion and hope, as well as on a sense of social justice as including a preferential option for the poor, Farley urges the churches to take a leadership role in reversing the ideologies of sexual inequality in which they have been complicit. While the principle of respect calls our attention to the inviolability of the individual, the need for autonomy and personal bodily integrity, the virtue of compassion unites us affectively to the needs of the sufferer, and calls us to act beneficently so as to

ameliorate his or her situation. Farley urges religious
traditions to advocate for the sharing of resources,
and a reordering of priorities in both national and
international communities.

Finally, however, Farley places moral discernment and decision in a complex and tragic situation
such as AIDS under the sign of paradox. "In the
deepest experiences of compassionate love, where
divine mercy is known and received and then given,
there is mystery unable to be encompassed by categories either of compassion or respect. In these
deepest experiences, however, the requirements of
compassion and the requirements of respect come
together in the requirements of a just and truthful
love." To some extent, respect can represent the
dignity of the person, and compassion the solidarity
of all in the common good. If so, then Farley's resort
to a "just and truthful love" in the case of insoluble
or ambiguously soluble quandaries can be compared
to McHugh's determination of the concrete meaning of the common good through practical, political
"middle-level" thinking and action. In other words,
it is a call for prudential reasoning about the proportionate good within the context at hand and the
limits of the possible.

The Catholic religious and theological response
to AIDS illustrates the practice-based nature of
moral reasoning, as well as the potential for social
practices based on Christian religious and moral
values to begin to enact changes for the common

good. Margaret Farley does not write from an ivory tower. Along with another Sister of Mercy, Eileen Hogan, she spearheaded three conferences for 2003-04, with the collaboration of women's religious congregations. These conferences aim to bring African women together with supporters from other continents, to share insights and develop responses to the AIDS crisis as it affects women. For example, monogamous married women often contract AIDS from husbands who work away from home for long periods. Those men often have sex with very poor women, who have no other way to earn what their children need to survive from day to day. And even if HIV-positive pregnant women can obtain the drug AZT and avoid passing the virus to their infants, they are usually forced to breast-feed because they cannot afford formula, and so run the risk again of passing on AIDS to their children. The project, "All-Africa Conference, Sister to Sister," has attracted cooperation and support from organizations as widespread as the Sisters of Mercy, USAID, Catholic Relief Services, CAFOD in the UK, Trocaire in Ireland, and the African Jesuit AIDS Network.[95]

In the United States alone, Catholic health care institutions and the Catholic Health Association have a tremendous ability to influence civil society, and state and federal policy at upper, local and "middle" levels. Almost fifteen percent of community hospitals in the United States, and hundreds of clinics and nursing homes, are operated under Catholic auspices, and twenty percent of all hospital beds are in Catholic institutions.[96] The effort to protect individual dignity and moral responsibility by dealing with moral issues by means of double effect, absolute norms focused in on individual "acts," categories of "intrinsically evil," and so on, has sometimes seemed at best a distraction from, and at worst a contradiction of, Catholic health care ministry's historic commitment to the poor and underserved. Yet the tensions between these two prongs continue to be worked out at the practical level, often by prudential middle-level solutions representing "the art of the possible." The same can be said of Catholic healthcare's need to partner with other health care organizations that do not subscribe to the full range of Catholic values, either personal or social.

When we turn to the international presence of the Catholic Church, especially regarding the AIDS crisis, the picture is even more striking. Catholic Relief Services sponsors AIDS projects that serve approximately two million people affected by HIV/AIDS in 31 countries, primarily Africa. CRS helps to build innovative community based programs that reduce transmission of HIV, and gives medical and social support to those suffering from AIDS. It also addresses the underlying causes of AIDS, including poverty, and the special vulnerabilities and burdens faced by women. According to the CRS website, its policy "calls for compassion, not simply sympathy. It calls us to affirm human dignity, responsibility and social justice, and most importantly, it exhorts us to seek effective means of addressing the AIDS crisis," in practical collaboration with "the poorest of the poor."[97] CRS efforts include a program for the HIV/AIDS orphan crisis in Uganda. They have built a network in Zimbabwe of 10 parish mission hospitals that have established AIDS Committees in every parish. Groups of volunteers visit and care for the sick, perform AIDS preventive education dramas, and help individuals generate income. In Senegal, a church HIV/AIDS service provides information for youth, women, prisoners and others, and provides counseling micro-credit for HIV positive people. These are only a few CRS activities, and many more could be offered from the work of the African Jesuit AIDS Network and Caritas International.

The Episcopal Conferences of Africa and Madagascar (SECAM), as well as national African bishops' conferences, have also taken up the cause of AIDS as an issue both of personal dignity and of the common good.[98] SECAM, for example, pledges to seek greater resources to address AIDS, and to identify ways in which parishes, dioceses, and national Episcopal conferences can develop program strategies. It commits itself to ensure that health, social, and educational services of the Church respond "appropriately" to the situation of persons with AIDS. Moreover, it pledges to "focus on the particular vulnerability of girls and the heavy burden on women in the context of the HIV pandemic in Africa."[99] Of course an ecclesiastical policy document does not immediately amount to effective programs "on the ground," especially where deeply rooted stigmas and discrimination against women are concerned. However, SECAM's position paper is important as a symbolic and moral advance toward implementing the "plan of action" it proposes.

Interestingly, in light of the major proportions of the crisis, and the bishops' clear awareness that the causes are multiple, they open the door to a more contextual approach to the morality of condom use. Typically forbidden by Catholic representatives on the grounds that condoms are a form of birth control, condom use to prevent disease is actually better understood as a medical or preventive measure, of which the prevention of conception during hetero-sexual intercourse is only an "unintended side effect" and a "lesser evil" justifiable by double effect.[100] It seems that the highly inflamed controversy over birth control and Church authority, rather than the actual morality of preventing HIV transmission using this means, has determined the resistance to the latter expressed by many Church spokesmen. Some Vatican representatives seem to recognize that the argument that condoms used for this purpose are "intrinsically evil" has little moral-theological basis. Hence, they are turning to the argument that allowing condom use will encourage promiscuity.[101] This, obviously, constitutes a concession that it is social contingencies, not intrinsic characteristics, which determine the morality of condoms, opening the door to the consideration of additional social consequences, like the prevention of a large number of deaths.

The African bishops, while stating in no uncertain terms that "the Church says NO to a culture of sexual disorders or loose morals," still assert that the ultimate rule governing condom use is conscience. "Love" might thus lead a person to use a condom to protect himself or herself or his or her partner.[102] Such a move opens the analysis of condoms to a context-based method. In light of SECAM's general social justice approach to AIDS, the invocation of "conscience" implies reference to social setting. It thus goes beyond just the immediate situation and characteristics of a single agent, to refer implicitly to the larger "common good" in which the person participates and on which the person's well-being is dependent. The bishops' position could also be seen as an example of a "middle-level," or practical, political, and institutional attempt to deal productively with a perplexing situation.

Conclusion

Bioethics in the era of globalization includes fair distribution of health care resources. Also in the broad picture are poverty, sexism, and racism, that make many more vulnerable to disease. Catholic bioethics must move outward from the principles

of traditional moral theology to embrace an ethics
of the common good.

The controversial nature of movement in this
direction is exemplified by earlier debates over the
principle of double effect and proportionalism. Proportionalism reflects the dawning social consciousness of moral theology. It was part of a revolution in
moral consciousness among Catholics. The critique
of double effect was prompted by the growing recognition that discernment, judgment, choice and
action, are part and parcel of a whole complex of
social relationships and responsibilities from which it
is very difficult to entirely extricate particular moral
choices. Yet the proportionalist critique has been
unable on its own to furnish the adequate social
analysis a bioethics of the common good requires.
During the past couple of decades, bioethics has been
brought increasingly within the purview of Catholic
social teaching. The responsibility to support human
life must now be placed in a global context. The
ethics of health care is more a matter of just resource
distribution than of individual choices to use or not
use readily available hi-tech interventions.

The AIDS pandemic is a particularly effective
and poignant illustration of this shift in bioethical
consciousness. AIDS requires that we address global
structures of wealth and poverty, as well as market-
based medicine and research, and cross-cultural
norms for sex and gender, especially those that result
in the oppression (and deaths) of women. Global

justice in health care seems like a utopian ideal. Even so, change in the patterns of access to health care is already occurring as the poor of the world claim their own right to participate in the common good, and as religiously committed advocates work to raise the sense of justice and level of altruism in privileged cultures. Structures and networks are developing locally and globally through which the participation of the poor and of those in solidarity with them is becoming more effective. Social inequities and conflicts between personal dignity and the common good will never be entirely eradicated. Yet bioethics in the new century is witnessing more creative, collaborative and prudential action to realize the human good "analogously" to the full good for which we hope. Hope for humanity's common good, and a vision of God as the ultimate good of all, can inspire the mutual "compassion and respect" required if persons and communities worldwide are to enjoy the basic good of health.

Notes

1 I thank Sarah Moses for doing research for this essay, and David Hollenbach and Margaret Farley for providing resources on the Catholic response to AIDS in Africa.

2 A major recent work on this tradition is David Hollenbach, S.J., *The Common Good and Christian Ethics* (Cambridge: Cambridge University Press, 2002).

3 James M. Gustafson, *The Contributions of Theology to Medical Ethics* (Milwaukee: Marquette University Theology Department, 1975) 29.

4 Ibid., 32.

5 Ibid., 35, 34.

6 Ibid., 87.

7 Ibid., 91.

8 Richard A. McCormick, S.J., *Ambiguity in Moral Choice* (Milwaukee: Marquette University Theology Department, 1973). This work is reprinted in its entirety in Richard A. McCormick, S.J., and Paul Ramsey, eds., *Doing Evil to Achieve Good: Moral Choice in Conflict Situations* (Chicago: Loyola University Press, 1978), from which citations shall be taken.

9 At the beginning of his lecture, McCormick states the conditions of double effect in the following terms:

> (1) The action is good or indifferent in itself; it is not morally evil. (2) The intention of the agent is upright, that is, the evil effect is sincerely not intended. (3) The evil effect must be equally immediate causally with the good effect, for otherwise it would be a means to the good effect and would be intended. (4) There must be a proportionately grave reason for allowing the evil to occur. If these conditions are fulfilled, the resultant evil was referred to as

an 'unintended byproduct' of the action, only indirectly voluntary and justified by the presence of a proportionately grave reason (7).

See also Gerald Kelly, S.J., *Medico-Moral Problems* (St. Louis: Catholic Health Association of the United States and Canada, 1957), 12-16.

10 A representative example is the case in which a pregnancy threatens the life of a woman. If she is given medicine to save her life, and it causes a "spontaneous" abortion as a side effect, the decision is permitted under double effect. However, if the fetus is directly removed by surgical abortion, also to save the mother's life, the action is described as direct and the death of the fetus is deemed "directly intended" and prohibited.

11 McCormick does not deny conflict, for example, of life against life (*Ambiguity in Moral Choice*, 47-48). But true conflicts of *moral* values are impossible. Moral values are values that have to do with the dignity and inviolability of the human person, and with the moral character of the person. Moral values are attributes of character and personal relationship like love, honesty, fidelity, and courage. A true moral conflict would be one in which one is required to "sin bravely," where the act is both a sin and morally required. (See McCormick, "A Commentary on the Commentaries," in *Doing Evil to Achieve Good*, 217, 222). A genuinely moral act cannot involve violations of moral virtues, such as "justice, truthfulness, fidelity" ("A Commentary," 223). "There is never a proportionate reason for sinning or intending another's sin" (ibid., 223).

Sometimes moral values are distinguished from "premoral" or "nonmoral" values like physical life, the integrity of physical processes, and material and social goods like food, shelter, education, and employment.

These can conflict, and sometimes one may have to be sacrificed for another, on the basis of some kind of measurement or estimate of the greatest good at stake. Obviously, in real human relationships, these types of values are closely connected. McCormick tends to think the good of life is the most fundamental, and most closely connected to the realization of moral goods (ibid., 216, 223, 228). Again, this has been a long and complicated discussion (ibid., 213-223). For a concise treatment, see Charles E. Curran, *The Catholic Moral Tradition Today: A Synthesis* (Washington, D.C.: Georgetown University Press, 1999) 152-60.

12 *Ambiguity in Moral Choice*, 9.

13 For this context, see Michael Manning, M.D., *Euthanasia and Physician-Assisted Suicide: Killing or Caring?* (New York/Mahwah: Paulist Press, 1998) 12-16.

14 These critics, who were not all saying exactly the same thing, came to be grouped loosely together and called "proportionalists," originally and primarily by adversaries who wanted to cast upon them the pall of utilitarianism. The resulting debate over proportionalism and double effect has been long, tireless, often tiresome, and sometimes vicious. For further discussion, see McCormick and Ramsey, eds., *Doing Evil to Achieve Good,* Charles E. Curran and Richard A. McCormick, S.J., eds., *Moral Norms and Catholic Tradition* (New York/Ramsey/Toronto: Paulist Press, 1979); Bernard Hoose, *Proportionalism: the American Debate and its European Roots* (Washington, D.C.: Georgetown University Press, 1987); William E. May, *Moral Absolutes* (Milwaukee: Marquette University Press, 1989); and Aline H. Kalbian, "Where Have All the Proportionalists Gone?," *Journal of Religious Ethics* 30 (2002) 3-22.

15 "A Commentary on the Commentaries," 222.

16 *Ambiguity in Moral Choice*, 46. McCormick insists that consequentialism "is certainly not what I mean by proportionate reason" ("A Commentary," 233).

17 Albert R. Jonsen and Stephen Toulmin, *The Abuse of Casuistry: A History of Moral Reasoning* (Los Angeles: University of California Press, 1988); James F. Keenan, S.J. and Thomas A. Shannon, *The Context of Casuistry* (Washington, D.C.: Georgetown University Press, 1995).

18 Aline Kalbian, "Where Have All the Proportionalists Gone?," *Journal of Religious Ethics* 30 (2002) 7. Kalbian draws on the work of James Keenan, S.J. and Edward Vacek, S.J., in developing this insight.

19 Ibid., 19.

20 Ibid., 15.

21 He also concludes that "indirect intention" is a way of distancing oneself morally from the evil that one's action may cause, as if to acknowledge that it represents a lamentable sacrifice in regard to human flourishing (*Ambiguity in Moral Choice*, 47-50).

22 John C. Ford, "The Morality of Obliteration Bombing," *Theological Studies* 5 (1944) 261-309.

23 "A Commentary," 232.

24 Ibid., 236-39

25 See Walter Rauschenbusch, *A Theology for the Social Gospel* (Nashville: Abingdon, 1945; originally published 1917).

26 Reinhold Niebuhr, *Moral Man and Immoral Society: A Study in Ethics and Politics* (New York: Scribner's, 1932, 1960).

27 See Gustavo Gutierrez, *A Theology of Liberation: History, Politics and Salvation* (Maryknoll NY: Orbis, 1973).

28 Ibid., 238.

29 Ibid., 257.

30 Ibid., 265.

31 May, *Moral Absolutes*. 49.

32 Ibid., 69.

33 Ibid., 67.

34 Ibid., 71.

35 Jonsen and Toulmin, *The Abuse of Casuistry*; Keenan and Shannon, *The Context of Casuistry*.

36 *Ambiguity in Moral Choice*, 50.

37 Gerald Kelly, S.J., *Medico-Moral Problems* (St. Louis: Catholic Health Association of the United States and Canada, 1957).

38 Gerald Kelly, S.J., "The Duty of Using Artificial Means of Preserving Life," *Theological Studies* 11 (1950) 207-208.

39 For a recent discussion of this principle, double effect, and other elements of the Catholic approach to death and dying, see Dolores L. Christie, *Last Rights: A Catholic Perspective on End-of-Life Decisions* (Lanham MD: Rowman and Littlefield, 2003).

40 "Richard A. McCormick, S.J., "To Save or Let Die: The Dilemma of Modern Medicine," *Journal of the American Medical Association* 229 (1974) 172-76. See also peter A. Clark, S.J., *To Treat or Not to Treat: The Ethical Methodology of Richard A. McCormick, S.J., as Applied to Treatment Decisions for Handicapped Newborns* (Omaha NE: Creighton University Press, 2003).

41 Ibid., 172.

42 James M. Gustafson, "Mongolism, Parental Desires, and the Right to Life," *Perspectives in Biology and Medicine* 16 (1973) 329-359.

43 McCormick cites this address from *Acta Apostolicae Sedis* 49 (1957) 1031-32. It is also available as Pope Pius XII, "Address to an International Congress of Anesthesiologists," *National Catholic Bioethics Quarterly* 2 (2002) 309-14.

44 Ibid., *Acta Apostolicae Sedis*, 311.

45 See Kelly, *Medico-Moral Problems*, 115-41; and the Sacred Congregation for the Doctrine of the Faith,

Declaration on Euthanasia (Boston: St. Paul Editions, 1980). According to the latter, "it will be possible to make a correct judgment as to the means by studying the type of treatment to be used, its degree of complexity or risk, its cost and the possibilities of using it, and comparing these elements with the result that can be expected, taking into account the state of the sick person and his or her physical and moral resources" (11).

46 On quality of life, see James J. Walter and Thomas A. Shannon, eds., *Quality of Life: The New Medical Dilemma* (New York and Mahwah NJ: Paulist, 1990).

47 Ibid., 174-75.

48 Ibid., 176.

49 John J. Paris, S.J. and Richard A. McCormick, S.J., "The Catholic Tradition on the Use of Nutrition and Fluids," *America* 156 (1987) 356-61; and, for a contrasting position, Joseph Torchia, O.P., "Artificial Hydration and Nutrition for the PVS Patient," *National Catholic Bioethics Quarterly* 3 (2003) 719-30. For an overview, see Christie, *Last Rights*, 119-33. Germain Grisez, one of the primary detractors of proportionalism, and certainly a defender of "pro-life" positions, does take cost and fairness specifically into account in deciding that comatose patients need not always be sustained indefinitely in intensive care facilities. See Germain Grisez, "Should Nutrition Be Provided to Permanently Comatose and Other Mentally Disabled Persons?," *Linacre Quarterly* 57 (1990) 41-42; and *The Way of the Lord Jesus, Vol. 2, Living a Christian Life* (Quincy IL: Franciscan Press, 1992) 531.

50 Richard A. McCormick, S.J, "Nutrition-Hydration: The New Euthanasia?," in *The Critical Calling: Reflections on Moral Dilemmas Since Vatican II* (Washington, D.C.: Georgetown University Press, 1989) 381.

51 Josephine M. Lumitao, "AIDS in the Developing World: The Case of the Philippines," in Angeles Tan Alora and Josephine M. Lumitao , eds., *Beyond Western Bioethics* (Washington, D.C.: Georgetown University Press, 2001) 85.

52 John S. Boswell, "Solidarity, Justice and power Sharing: Patterns and Policies," in J.S. Boswell, F. P. McHugh, J. Verstraeten,eds. *Catholic Social Thought: Twilight or Renaissance?* (Leuven: Leuven University Press, 2000) 103-04. See also Francis P. McHugh, "Muddle or Middle-Level? A Place for Natural law in Catholic Social Thought," in the same volume, 51.

53 See Kelly, *Medico-Moral Problems*, 128-141.

54 See United States Bishops, "Resolution on Health Care Reform," *Origins* 23 (1993) 98-102; and Catholic Hospital Association, *With Justice for All? The Ethics of Health Care Rationing* (St, Louis MO: Catholic Health Association, 1991).

55 Committee on Doctrine of the National Conference of Catholic Bishops, *Ethical and Religious Directives for Catholic Health Facilities* (Washington, D.C.: U.S. Catholic Conference, 1971, revised 1975) 1.

56 Committee on Doctrine of the National Conference of Catholic Bishops, *Ethical and Religious Directives for Catholic Health Care Services*, Fourth Edition (Washington, D.C.: United States Catholic Conference, 2001) 1-2; accessed at *http://www.usccb.org/bishops/directives. htm*.

57 Ibid., 12.

58 Ibid., 10.

59 John Paul II, *Address to the Pontifical Academy for Life*, 2003, as cited in Catholic Health Association of the United States, *Genetics, Science, and the Church: A Synopsis of Catholic Church Teachings on Science and Genetics* (St. Louis: Catholic Health Association of the

United States, 2003) 7; accessed at the CHA website *(http://www.chausa.org)*.

60 Philip S. Keane, S.S., *Catholicism and Health Care Justice: Problems, Potential And Solutions* (New York/ Mahwah: Paulist Press, 2002) 190-91.

61 Clarke E. Cochran and David Carroll Cochran, *Catholics, Politics, & Public Policy: Beyond Left and Right* (Maryknoll, NY: Orbis Books, 2003) 50.

62 Ibid., 52.

63 See Keane, *Catholicism and Health-Care Justice*, 23-25; Cochrans, *Catholics, Politics…*, 8; and B. Andrew Lustig, "Health Care in the Light of Catholic Teaching," in *Secular Bioethics in Theological Perspective*, ed. Earl E. Shelp (Boston: Kluwer, 1996) 32, 34-35.

64 Ibid., 34-35.

65 For further discussion, see David Barnard, "In the High Court of South Africa: Case No. 4138/98: The Global Politics of Access to Low-Cost AIDS Drugs in Poor Countries," *Kennedy Institute of Ethics Journal* 12 (2002) 159-74; and Lisa Sowle Cahill, "Biotech and Justice: Catching Up with the Real World Order," *Hastings Center Report* 33 (2003) 39-42. An editorial, "AIDS: The Ever-Growing Scourge," *America* 189 (August 4-11, 2003) 3, reviews the status of international donations to fight AIDS. See also a discussion of AIDS and patenting in Maura A. Ryan, "Beyond a Western Bioethics," to appear in *Theological Studies* 63/1 (2004), read in manuscript.

66 World Health Organization, *World Health Report 2003—Shaping the Future*. The December 2003 report and a press release, "Urgent Work Needed to Rebuild Health Care Systems," were accessed at the WHO website, *http://www.who.int*. The statistics to follow were drawn from this release and Colin Nickerson, "Amid the Death, New Hope: From Education to Vaccines, a

Drive to Halt Malaria Takes Off," *Boston Sunday Globe*, December 28, 2003, A1, A18-19.

67 This last statistic comes from the Southern Africa Catholic Bishops' Conference, as cited in "Signs of the Times," *America* 189 (December 15, 2003) 4.

68 Norman Daniels, Bruce P. Kennedy, and Ichiro Kawachi, "Why Social Justice is Good for Our Health: The Social Determinants of Health Inequalities," *Daedalus* 128 (1999) 215-251. See also, Giovanni Berlinguer, "Bioethics, Power and Injustice," in Volnei Garrafa and Leo Pessini, eds., *Bioetica: Poder e Injustica* (Sao Paulo, Brasil: Edicioes Loyola, 2003) 45-58.

69 Veena Das, ""Public Good, Ethics, and Everyday life: Beyond the Boundaries of Bioethics," *Daedalus* 128 (1999) 99-133.

70 For an analysis and overview of this direction of critique and its consequences, see Ryan, "Beyond a Western Bioethics." See also Godfrey B. Tangwa, "Globalisation or Westernisation? Ethical Concerns in the Whole Bio-Business," *Bioethics* 13 (1999) 218-26; Angeles Tan Alora and Josephine M. Lumitao, "An Introduction to an Authentically Non-Western Bioethics," *Beyond a Western Bioethics*, 3-19. Ryan cites Tangwa and gives a substantial discussion of the Alora/Lumitao volume.

71 Ibid., 8.

72 Josephine M. Lumitao, ""Death and Dying," in *Beyond Western Bioethics*, 97.

73 Ibid., 99.

74 Ibid., 97.

75The emergence of pastoral care and spirituality as a more prominent aspect of bioethics is illustrated by works that combine moral-theological analysis with pastoral concerns, liturgical models, and advice on matters such as overcoming disagreement among family members and composing advance directives. See Thomas A. Shannon and Charles N. Faso, O.F.M., *Let Them Go*

Free: A Family Prayer Service to Assist in the Withdrawal of Life Support Systems (Kansas City: Sheed and Ward, 1985); Catholic Health Association, *Care of the Dying: A Catholic Perspective* (St. Louis: Catholic Health Association, 1993); and Christie, *Last Rights*.

76 See, for example, Daniel Callahan, *Setting Limits: Medical Goals in an Aging Society* New York and London: Simon and Schuster, 1987).

77 Jacques Maritain, (Notre Dame IN: University of Notre Dame Press, 1947) 51.

78 Sharon LaFraniere, "AIDS Patients in Zambia Face Stark Choices," *New York Times*, October 11, 2003, A1.

79 Boswell, "Solidarity," 105.

80 John Paul II, *Sollicitudo Rei Socialis* (1987), in David J. O'Brien and Thomas A. Shannon, eds., *Catholic Social Thought: The Documentary Heritage* (Maryknoll, NY: Orbis, 1998) 421.

81 Ibid., 422.

82 Boswell, "Solidarity," 103-04.

83 Ibid., 106-07

84 Ibid., 107.

85 Ibid., 111.

86 Ibid., 112, 114.

87 Ryan, "Beyond a Western Bioethics?"

88 McHugh, "Muddle or Middle-Level?," 51.

89 See Kenneth Overberg, S.J., ed., *AIDS, Ethics and Religion: Embracing a World of Suffering* (Maryknoll NY: Orbis, 1994); and James F. Keenan, S.J., ed., *Catholic Ethicists on HIV/AIDS Prevention* (New York and London: Continuum, 2000).

90 See Diana Bader, O.P. and Elizabeth McMillan, R.S.M., *AIDS: Ethical Guidelines for Healthcare Providers*, first edition revised (St. Louis MO: Catholic Health Association of the United States, 1989).

91 For a more thorough discussion, see Lisa Sowle Cahill, "Genetics, Ethics, and Feminist Theology: Some Recent Directions," *Journal of Feminist Studies in Religion* (2002) 53-77.

92 Margaret A. Farley, "Issues in Contemporary Christian Ethics: The Choice of Death in a Medical Context," *The Santa Clara Lectures* (Santa Clara CA: Santa Clara University,1993) 13.

93 Margaret A. Farley, *Compassionate Respect: A Feminist Approach to Medical Ethics and Other Questions* (New York/Mahwah: Paulist, 2002).

94 Ibid., 14-15.

95 See George M. Anderson, "Sister-to-Sister: A New Approach to AIDS in Africa," *America* 189 (August 4-11, 2003) 16-17.

96 Cochrans, *Catholics, Politics and Public Policy*, 50.

97 Accessed at the CRS website, *http://www.catholicrelief. org*.

98 For a summary, see the unsigned "Signs of the Times" feature, *America* 189 (December 15, 2003) 4.

99 SECAM, ""The Church in Africa in Face of the HIV/ AIDS Pandemic," issued by SECAM, Dakar, Senegal, 7/10/03, and distributed by Kenya Episcopal Conference, Nairobi, December 2003.

100 An overview of recent clashes in this debate is offered in "Signs of the Times," *America* 190 (January 5-12, 2004) 4-5. See also Kenneth R. Overberg, S.J., "AIDS: A Worsening Crisis Challenges Society and Religion," in *AIDS, Ethics & Religion*, 1-9; and Jon D. Fuller, S.J., and James F. Keenan, S.J., "Introduction: At the End of the First Generation of HIV Prevention," in *Catholic Ethicists*, 21-38.

101 "Signs of the Times" (January 5-12, 2004) 4.

102 SECAM, *Our Prayer for You Is Always Full of Hope* (Accra, Ghana: SECAM Secretariat, 2003) 2-73.

The Père Marquette Lectures in Theology

1969 *The Authority for Authority*
Quentin Quesnell

1970 *Mystery and Truth*
John Macquarrie

1971 *Doctrinal Pluralism*
Bernard Lonergan, S.J.

1972 *Infallibility*
George A. Lindbeck

1973 *Ambiguity in Moral Choice*
Richard A. McCormick, S.J.

1974 *Church Membership as a Catholic and Ecumenical Problem*
Avery Dulles, S.J.

1975 *The Contributions of Theology to Medical Ethics*
James Gustafson

1976 *Religious Values in an Age of Violence*
Rabbi Marc Tannenbaum
Director of National Interreligious Affairs

1977 *Truth Beyond Relativism: Karl Mannheim's Sociology of Knowledge*
Gregory Baum

1978 *A Theology of 'Uncreated Energies'*
George A. Maloney, S.J.
John XXIII Center for Eastern Christian Studies

1980 *Method in Theology: An Organon For Our Time*
Frederick E. Crowe, S.J.

THE PÈRE MARQUETTE LECTURES IN THEOLOGY

1981 *Catholics in the Promised Land of the Saints*
James Hennesey, S.J.

1982 *Whose Experience Counts in Theological Reflection?*
Monika Hellwig

1983 *The Theology and Setting of Discipleship in the Gospel of Mark*
John R. Donahue, S.J.

1984 *Should War be Eliminated? Philosophical and Theological Investigations*
Stanley Hauerwas

1985 *From Vision to Legislation: From the Council to a Code of Laws*
Ladislas M. Orsy, S.J.

1986 *Revelation and Violence: A Study in Contextualization*
Walter Brueggemann
Eden Theological Seminary

1987 *Nova et Vetera: The Theology of Tradition in American Catholicism*
Gerald Fogarty

1988 *The Christian Understanding of Freedom and the History of Freedom in the Modern Era: The Meeting and Confrontation Between Christianity and the Modern Era in a Postmodern Situation*
Walter Kasper

1989 *Moral Absolutes: Catholic Tradition, Current Trends, and the Truth*
William F. May

1990 *Is Mark's Gospel a Life of Jesus? The Question of Genre*
Adela Yarbro Collins

THE PÈRE MARQUETTE LECTURES IN THEOLOGY

THE PÈRE MARQUETTE LECTURES IN THEOLOGY

About the Père Marquette Lecture Series

The Annual Père Marquette Lecture Series began at Marquette University in the Spring of 1969. Ideal for classroom use, library additions, or private collections, the Père Marquette Lecture Series has received international acceptance by scholars, universities, and libraries. Hardbound in blue cloth with gold stamped covers. Uniform style and price ($15 each). Some reprints with soft covers. Regular reprinting keeps all volumes available. Ordering information (purchase orders, checks, and major credit cards accepted):

Marquette University Press
1444 U.S. Route 42
P.O. Box 388
Ashland OH 44903

Order Toll-Free (800) 247-6553
fax: (419) 281 6883

Editorial Address:

Dr. Andrew Tallon, Director
Marquette University Press
Box 1881
Milwaukee WI 53201-1881

phone:	(414) 288-7298
fax:	(414) 288-3300
internet:	andrew.tallon@marquette.edu
web:	www.marquette.edu/mupress/

The Père Marquette Lectures in Theology

ISBN 0-87462-584-X